Zen Cookery

previously published as
The First Macrobiotic Cookbook

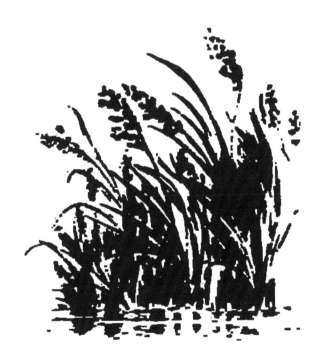

George Ohsawa Macrobiotic Foundation
Chico, California

Books by George Ohsawa in English include: *Acupuncture and the Philosophy of the Far East; Atomic Age and the Philosophy of the Far East;* Book of Judo; *Cancer and the Philosophy of the Far East; Essential Ohsawa; Gandhi, the Eternal Youth; Jack and Mitie; Macrobiotic Guidebook for Living; Macrobiotics: An Invitation to Health and Happiness; Order of the Universe; Philosophy of Oriental Medicine; Practical Guide to Far Eastern Macrobiotic Medicine; Unique Principle; You Are All Sanpaku;* and *Zen Macrobiotics.* Contact the publisher at the address below for a complete list of available titles.

This book is made possible through a contribution from Ayrin Kasala.

Keyboarding by Alice Salinero
Proofreading/editing by Kathy Keller
Text layout and design by Carl Ferré
Cover design by Carl Campbell

First Edition	1964
Second Edition	1984
Third Edition	1985
Current Printing: edited and reformatted	2012 Sep 1

© copyright 1985, 1984 by
George Ohsawa Macrobiotic Foundation
   PO Box 3998, Chico, California 95927-3998
   530-566-9765; fax 530-566-9768; *gomf@earthlink.net*
   www.ohsawamacrobiotics.com

Published with the help of East West Center for Macrobiotics
   www.eastwestmacrobiotics.com

ISBN 978-0-918860-68-2

Contents

We express our deep appreciation to George and Lima Ohsawa, who spread macrobiotics around the world and wrote the original manuscript that inspired Zen Cookery. The Ohsawas' students, Herman and Cornellia Aihara, continued to spread macrobiotic philosophy and diet in the United States. This book is largely the result of Cornellia's teaching and help with recipe revisions and Herman's twenty-five years of macrobiotic publishing.

As with any book having a long and varied history, many people have put their time, talents, and energy into the various editions of this book and, thus, have an influence on the present work. We wish to thank each one.

Many of the original recipes were furnished by Joanne Hirsh, Dorothy Salant, Nina Bauman, Penny Smith, Betty Kennedy, and Jane Andrews. Editing and coordination of the first edition was by Teal Nichols, and the second edition by Shayne Oles. Kevin Meutsch, Annette Hafer, Sandy Rothman, Chris Lentz, and Julie Morris contributed to the second edition.

Finally, we thank Carl Ferré for designing and producing this third edition; Laurel Ruggles for editing and revising recipes with the assistance of Cornellia Aihara; Sylvia Zuck for typesetting; and Lily Toppenberg for cover art.

George Ohsawa Macrobiotic Foundation

Preface

Soon after George Ohsawa came to the United States to promote macrobiotics in 1959 and published *Zen Macrobiotics* in 1960. This book in its original form included recipes for macrobiotic cooking. Although the number of macrobiotic students increased rapidly because of his interesting lectures and charisma, the much needed editing of the recipes for clearer instructions and measurements was not realized until later.

In 1961, on Ohsawa's advice, thirteen macrobiotic families, numbering thirty-four people, left New York City and moved to a small town in Northern California named Chico. The following year, all the adult members of the group started the first macrobiotic food distributing company, Chico-San, Inc.

Because nobody on the West Coast had heard of macrobiotic foods, one of the first jobs for the Chico-San founders was educating people in the macrobiotic philosophy, diet, and cooking. A committee for the teaching of macrobiotic cooking was formed by the women of the group who began by separating the cooking section from *Zen Macrobiotics* and gathering recipes among themselves. Thus, Chico-San, under the name of the Ohsawa Foundation of Chico, published the first macrobiotic cookbook, *Zen Cookery*, in 1964.

The book sold very well for eleven years. It was out of print from 1975 until 1984, when the George Ohsawa Macrobiotic Foundation published the book under a new title, *The First Macrobiotic Cookbook*. The 1985 edition was completely revised and corrected; however, the original outline and numbering system have been retained.

We and the Foundation's staff are happy to be publishing this revised edition after many corrections of recipes, instructions, and cooking styles. We are very proud of this book and hope that not only will it help people to cook macrobiotic meals but also that it will inspire the macrobiotic spirit and movement in this country. After all, this is not just a cookbook but a cornerstone of macrobiotic life in the United States.

– Cornellia and Herman Aihara
July, 1985

Recollections
of the early 1960s

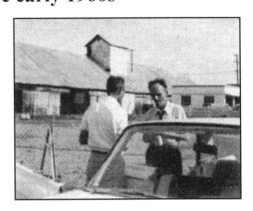

Bill Salant, Al Bauman, and Herman Aihara (not in picture) stop for refreshment on their exploration of the Sacramento Valley area prior to the cross-country move.

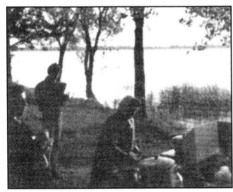

On the road: Cornellia Aihara preparing breakfast for 36 hungry people at a scenic spot near Lincoln, Nebraska, on the way to California.

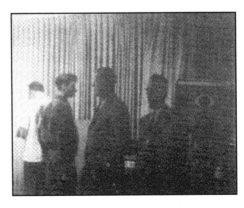

CBS News is on hand to greet the travellers upon their arrival in Chico. Later, a 'Welcome to Chico' dinner was sponsored by the town.

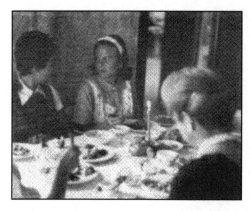

Joanne Hirsh (left) with Teal Nichols (center), editor of the first edition of *Zen Cookery*.

Shayne Oles, editor of *The New Zen Cookery*, with husband Lou (left) and Junsei Yamazaki.

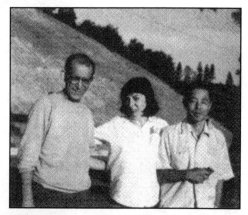

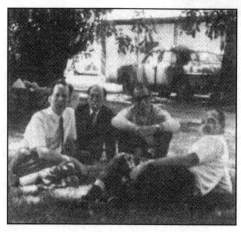

Jacques deLangre, Tommy Nakayama, Lou Oles, and Bob Kennedy relaxing in front of Herman and Cornellia Aihara's home.

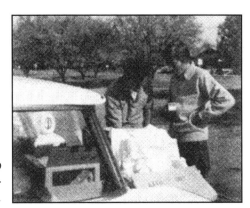

Herman Aihara rings up a sale at the first 'Chico-San'—the tailgate of his car.

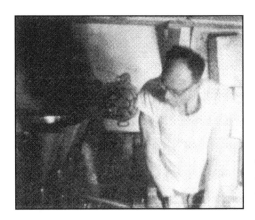

Irv Hirsh getting a workout on the first rice cake machine (modified) in the United States.

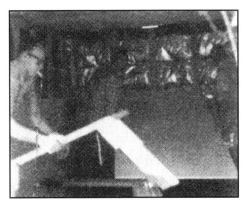

Construction underway on a koji room at the Chico-San facility in Chico.

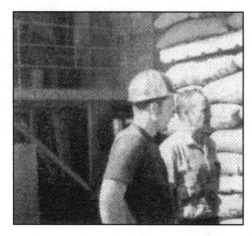

Bob Kennedy (right), president of Chico-San until its sale in 1985, standing in front of a new shipment of organic rice.

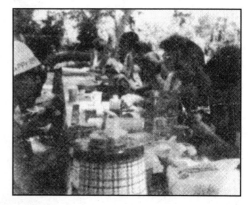

Meal time at the premier Chico picnic; still held annually at Hooker Oak Park.

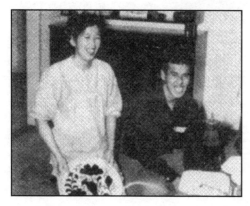

Herman and Cornellia Aihara, hosting the 1964 New Year's Day celebration.

Grains

Rice: Whole, unpolished, brown rice should be used because it contains all the vitamins and minerals of the rice. Short grain rice is recommended for general use in temperate climates. All grains should be organically grown.

1. Rice

A. Pressure Cooked Rice

1 cup rice
1¼ cups water
Pinch of salt

Wash rice thoroughly in cold water. Place ingredients in a pressure cooker and bring to full pressure. Lower heat and cook 40 to 45 minutes. Turn off heat and allow pressure to return to normal. Let stand for 10 to 20 minutes. Mix rice thoroughly before serving. Note: For larger amounts of rice, reduce proportion of liquid slightly.

B. Boiled Rice

1 cup rice
2 cups water
Pinch of salt

Wash rice thoroughly in cold water. Bring to a boil in heavy pot, lower flame, and simmer for one hour or until liquid is absorbed. Mix thoroughly before serving.

C. Baked Rice

2 cups rice
4 cups boiling water
⅛ tsp salt
1 tsp soy sauce

Wash rice thoroughly in cold water. In a dry pan, roast rice until it is golden and begins to pop. Place ingredients in a covered casserole and bake for 45 minutes in a 350-degree oven.

2. Rice with Soy Sauce

Using any cooking method, add 1 tablespoon soy sauce for each cup of rice and omit salt. Cook as directed.

3. Rice with Azuki Beans

3 cups rice
⅓ cup azuki beans
4½ cups water
½ tsp salt

Wash rice and azuki beans. Place ingredients in pressure cooker and bring to full pressure. Lower heat and cook 45 minutes. Turn off heat and allow pressure to return to normal. Let stand 10 minutes. Remove cover and mix before serving.

Variation: Using 6 cups of water, bring azuki beans to a boil in a heavy pot. Add rice and salt and cook over low heat about 1 hour, or until water is absorbed.

4. Rice and Azuki Pudding

1 cup rice
¼ cup azuki beans
¼ tsp salt
5 to 6 cups water

Wash rice and azuki beans. Pressure cook ingredients together 45 minutes over low heat. Allow pressure to return to normal. Mix before serving.

Variation: Using 12 cups water, bring azuki beans and rice to a boil in a heavy pot. Simmer 1 hour or until beans are soft. Add salt and simmer a few minutes longer. Mix before serving.

5. Vegetables and Rice

Cooked rice
Cooked vegetables, nitsuke

To rice cooked by any method, add 5-10 percent cooked vegetables.

6. Fried Rice

Prepare Vegetables and Rice (5). Pan fry in a small amount of oil. Add soy sauce to taste.

7. Sesame Rice

3 cups cooked rice
⅓ cup unhulled sesame seeds

Roast sesame seeds in a dry pan. Mix with cooked rice.

8. Chestnut Rice

3 cups rice
½ cup fresh or dried chestnuts
¼ tsp salt
4½ cups water

Wash rice. Place ingredients in pressure cooker and bring to full pressure. Lower heat and cook 45 minutes, Turn off heat and allow pressure to return to normal. Let stand 10 minutes. Mix before serving.

Variation: Using 6 cups of water, bring chestnuts to a boil in a heavy pot. Add rice and salt and cook over low heat about 1 hour, or until water is absorbed.

9. Rice with Chickpeas

3 cups rice
⅓ cup chickpeas
4½ cups water
½ tsp salt

Wash rice and chickpeas. Pressure cook ingredients together over low heat for 45 minutes. Allow pressure to return to normal. Mix before serving.

Variation: Prepare Chickpeas and Onions (103 A) and serve over cooked rice.

10. Rice Mold

2 carrots, cut in matchsticks
2 lotus roots, thinly sliced
¼ bunch watercress, chopped
2 beaten eggs (optional)
3 cups cooked rice

Sauté each vegetable separately in a small amount of sesame oil with a pinch of salt. Add a little water to cover the bottom of the pan; cover and cook all the vegetables together over low heat until done. Add soy sauce to taste. Fry beaten eggs in a thin layer and shred. Arrange vegetables and egg attractively in a rectangular baking dish. On top of this, press down rice to a 2-inch thickness. Invert over a platter and unmold. Cut into serving portions.

11. Rice Croquettes

A. Pan Fried Croquettes
        2 cups cooked rice
        ½ cup leftover rice cream cereal (16A, B, or C)
        Whole wheat flour
        3 Tbsp oil
        1 egg (optional)

Mix rice and rice cream cereal. Form into patties. Dip first in beaten egg, then in flour. Pan fry in oil until crisp.

B. Deep Fried Croquettes
        2 cups cooked rice
        ½ carrot, chopped or grated
        1 small onion, chopped
        2 cabbage leaves, chopped
        ½ tsp salt
        ½ cup whole wheat flour
        Oil for deep frying

Mix vegetables, salt, and rice with enough whole wheat flour and water to make it easy to form patties that hold together. Deep fry until crisp. Test to determine that the center is cooked.

12. Rice Pie
        Cooked vegetables
        Cooked rice
        Soy sauce
        Béchamel Sauce (159 B)
        Pastry (253)

Add 10 to 20 percent cooked vegetables to cooked rice. Mix with béchamel sauce. Soy sauce may be added to taste. Fit pastry to pie pan. Fill with the rice mixture. Cover with top crust and bake 45 minutes in a 350-degree oven or until the crust is golden brown.

13. Rice Balls

> Cooked rice
> Small bowl of salted water (5 percent salt)

Dip hands in cold salted water. Take about 2 tablespoons cooked rice and press to form round or triangular shaped balls.

Variations:

Place a small piece of Japanese salted plum (umeboshi) in the center of each ball. The flavor is delicious and the rice balls will not spoil for a few days when not refrigerated, even in the summer. Good for traveling.

Place 2 or 3 pieces of Kombu in Soy Sauce (111) in the center of each rice ball.

Use nori seaweed to partially wrap each rice ball, patting nori at the edges until it adheres.

Sprinkle rice balls with small amount of roasted sesame seeds or gomashio.

Prepare Sesame Rice (7) and form into balls.

Prepare Azuki Rice (3) and form into balls

Prepare Rice and Vegetables (5) and form into balls.

Deep fry rice balls until golden.

14. Rice Cereals

A. Pressure Cooked Rice Porridge

> 1 cup rice
> 4 cups water
> ¼ tsp salt

Wash rice. Pressure cook ingredients 45 minutes. Allow pressure to return to normal.

B. Boiled Rice Porridge

> 1 cup rice
> 5 cups water
> ¼ tsp salt

Wash rice. Bring ingredients to a boil in a heavy pot. Lower heat and simmer 1 hour or longer.

C. Rice Porridge with Soy Sauce

Prepare porridge by any method using 1 tablespoon soy sauce per cup of rice, omitting salt.

D. Rice Porridge with Miso
    2 cups rice
    12 cups water
    ¼ cup miso

Wash rice. Pressure cook all ingredients 45 minutes over low heat or bring to a boil in heavy pot and simmer 1 hour or longer.
    Variations:
    Add miso soup to cooked rice and cook to desired consistency.
    Add a piece of baked or fried mochi when serving.

15. Special Rice Cream
    1 cup rice
    5 cups water
    ¼ tsp salt

Wash rice and roast in a heavy dry pan, stirring constantly until golden. Add water and salt. Bring to a boil and simmer 1 hour. Strain, or purée in a food mill.

16. Rice Cream Powder
    To prepare powder, wash rice and roast in a dry pan until golden. Put through flour mill or blend at high speed in a blender until it is like powder. Rice cream powder may be purchased but it is better when freshly made.

A. Pressure Cooked Rice Cream
    1 cup rice cream powder
    3½ to 4 cups boiling water
    ¼ tsp salt

Roast rice cream powder until there is a nut-like fragrance. Add water gradually, stirring constantly to prevent lumping. Add salt. Bring to full pressure. Lower heat and cook 20 minutes. Turn off heat and allow pressure to return to normal. Let stand 10 to 20 minutes. Mix thoroughly before serving.

B. Boiled Rice Cream
    1 cup rice cream powder
    4 cups boiling water
    ¼ tsp salt

Roast rice cream powder until fragrant; add water and salt. Bring to a boil, lower flame and simmer for 30 to 45 minutes. Mix thoroughly before serving.

C. Thick Rice Cream
   1 cup rice cream
   2 cups boiling water
   ¼ tsp salt

Roast rice cream powder until fragrant. Bring to sink and add ¼ teaspoon salt and 1 cup boiling water. Mix quickly and thoroughly. It will resemble a heavy dough-like mixture. To the pan, add the second cup of boiling water, pushing aside the dough so that the water covers the bottom of the pan forming a bed for the dough to steam on. Cover tightly and cook over low heat for 30 to 45 minutes. Mix thoroughly before serving.

17. Wheat Cream
   1 cup whole wheat flour or graham flour
   ¼ tsp salt
   4 cups boiling water

Roast flour in a heavy dry pan. Add water and salt. Bring to a boil and simmer 30 to 45 minutes. Mix before serving.

18. Popped Rice
   3 cups brown rice or sweet brown rice
   ¼ cup salt
   Water to cover

Wash rice and soak in water to cover for 48 hours. Drain and rinse. Add fresh water and the salt and soak another 24 hours. Drain. In a hot pan, roast rice, ½ cup at a time, stirring constantly until the rice pops and can be chewed easily.

19. Rice Canapes (Sushi)
   Raw tuna
   Eggs
   Clams
   Cooked rice
   Orange juice
   Soy sauce
   Grated ginger

Slice tuna into thin pieces. Beat eggs and make an omelette about ¼-inch thick. Cut into pieces the same size as tuna. Take clams out of shells. Boil in soy sauce for a few minutes. Mix about 1 tablespoon orange juice with each cup of rice. Let rice cool. Place a heaping tablespoon of rice in palm of left hand; with the first two fingers of the right hand, shape rice into cylinder shapes with slightly flattened top surfaces. Place either tuna, egg, or clams on each of the cylinders. Press down with fingers. Arrange attractively on platter. Serve with soy sauce to which a little grated ginger has been added.

20. Sushi Mold

>   Raw tuna
>   Cooked rice
>   Orange juice
>   Lotus root, thinly sliced
>   Carrots, cut in matchsticks
>   Eggs
>   Soy Sauce

Slice tuna into thin pieces. Mix about 1 tablespoon orange juice with each cup of rice. Let rice cool. Cook vegetables separately; sauté covered in a small amount of oil with a pinch of salt, add a small amount of water, cover and cook until done. Beat eggs and make an omelette about ¼-inch thick. Cut into pieces the same size as tuna. Wet a rectangular, shallow mold. Arrange fish, fried egg, and vegetables attractively. Cover with about 1 inch of rice. Press down, invert over platter, and unmold. Slice into rectangular pieces. Serve with soy sauce.

Variation: Place prepared rice in individual serving dishes and arrange fish, vegetables, and egg over rice.

21. Buckwheat Groats

>   1 cup raw buckwheat groats
>   2 cups boiling water
>   ¼ tsp salt
>   ¼ tsp oil

Wash and drain groats. Sauté in oil 5 minutes, stirring constantly. Add salt and boiling water. Cover and simmer for 20 minutes. Serve with Onion Nitsuke (65) or Onion Sauce (80G).

22. Baked Buckwheat Groats

Prepare Buckwheat Groats (21). Place cooked groats in a casserole and bake in a 350-degree oven for 45 minutes or until the top turns brown. Serve with any vegetable sauce.

23. Buckwheat Croquettes

> ½ cup buckwheat groats
> ¼ tsp oil
> ¼ tsp salt
> 1 cup boiling water
> 1 large onion, chopped
> Oil for deep frying
> ½ cup whole wheat pastry flour
> ¼ cup water

Sauté groats in oil for 5 minutes, stirring constantly. Add salt and boiling water. Cover and simmer for 20 minutes. Sauté onions in oil and mix with groats. Add enough whole wheat flour and water to make the dough a consistency which will allow you to roll small balls that will hold together. Roll each ball in whole wheat flour and deep fry until outside is crisp. Cut one in half to check if the center is cooked.

Variations:

Pan fry by making the batter thinner and dropping by spoon into an oiled skillet.

Pour Light Béchamel Sauce (159 B) over the fried croquettes.

24. Buckwheat Casserole

> 1 cup buckwheat groats
> 2 cups water
> ½ tsp salt
> 8 whole cabbage leaves
> 2 eggs, beaten (optional)

Mix buckwheat with water and salt. Oil a heavy iron casserole. Place a leaf of cabbage on the bottom, pour a layer of buckwheat mixture over this, and then a layer of egg, and top it off with another cabbage leaf. Alternate in this manner, having a cabbage leaf on top. Cover and bake in a 350-degree oven for 1½ hours. Remove from the pan by inverting over a platter. Cut at the table while still hot. Or serve directly from the casserole. Serve with soy sauce.

25. Thick Buckwheat Cream

    1 cup buckwheat flour
    ⅛ tsp salt
    2 cups boiling water
    Scallions
    Soy sauce

Roast buckwheat flour and salt for a few minutes in a dry pan. Add boiling water and mix vigorously. Turn off heat and serve immediately. Serve with chopped scallions and soy sauce.

26. Buckwheat Cream

    2 heaping Tbsp buckwheat flour
    1 tsp oil
    1 to 2 cups water
    ⅛ tsp salt
    Croutons

Sauté flour in oil for a few minutes. Add water and salt and boil until thickened. Pour into soup bowls and serve with croutons.
    Variation: Sauté onions and add to the cream while it is cooking.

27. Fried Buckwheat

    1 cup buckwheat flour
    1½ cups boiling water
    ¼ tsp salt

Mix ingredients together and drop by spoon into hot oil. Fry until outside is crisp.
    Variations:
    Add minced onion to batter.
    Make batter thinner by adding more water. Fry as thin crepes in lightly oiled, heated skillet.

28. Homemade Buckwheat Noodles

    1 lb buckwheat flour
    1 egg
    1 tsp salt
    ¾ cup boiling water

Mix all ingredients and knead well until smooth and shiny. Roll out to a thickness of one-tenth inch, roll up and slice as thinly as possible. Drop noodles into boiling water and cook until done. Drain and separate by pouring cold water over them and drain in a colander.

29. Millet

    2 cups millet
    6 cups boiling water
    ½ tsp salt

Wash millet. If desired, roast millet in pan for 5 to 10 minutes or until color turns, and it has a nut-like fragrance. Add water and salt and pressure cook for 30 minutes. Serve with cooked vegetables or Miso Sauce (204).

    Variation: Roast millet until fragrant. Using 8 cups water, boil millet and salt for 30 minutes.

30. Browned Millet with Onions

    1 cup millet
    1 Tbsp oil
    ½ cup onions, chopped
    ¼ tsp salt
    4 cups boiling water

Place the millet in a dry, heavy iron skillet or pot and brown slightly, stirring constantly. When it is turning color and has a nutty fragrance, remove from the pan temporarily. In this same skillet add oil and sauté onions until transparent. Add browned millet, salt and boiling water. Cover tightly and simmer for 25 to 30 minutes. Continue stirring occasionally.

31. Millet and Vegetables

    2 cups millet
    2 cups onions, carrot, squash; chopped
    2 tsp oil
    6 cups boiling water
    ½ tsp salt

Roast millet in a heavy, dry pan until fragrant and slightly browned. Sauté vegetables in oil. Combine millet, vegetables, water and salt. Bring to a boil and simmer 30 minutes.

32. Rolled Oats

> 2 cups rolled oats
> 4 to 5 cups water
> ¼ to ½ tsp salt

Roast oats until fragrant. Cool. Add 2 cups cold water and salt. Bring to boil, then add 2 to 3 more cups cold water. Bring to a boil again, then simmer for one hour or until desired consistency. Stir occasionally. Serve with sesame salt. This cereal can be cooked the night before or slowly simmered overnight in a double boiler on a low flame.

33. Cracked Wheat with Onions

> 2 cups cracked wheat
> 2 onions, chopped
> 1 Tbsp oil
> ¼ to ½ tsp salt
> 6 cups boiling water

Brown wheat in frying pan slowly until slightly colored and fragrant. Sauté onions in oil. Combine wheat, onions, salt, and boiling water. Cover and simmer for one hour, stirring occasionally. Add more water if necessary.

Variation: Add a pinch of thyme, basil, or garlic.

34. Bulghur

> 1 cup bulghur
> 1 tsp oil
> 2 cups boiling water
> ¼ tsp salt

Sauté bulghur in oil 5 minutes, stirring constantly. Add boiling water and salt and simmer 10 minutes.

Variation: Cook minced onions or carrots with bulghur.

35. Cornmeal Cereal

> 1 cup cornmeal
> ⅛ tsp oil (optional)
> ¼ tsp salt
> 3 to 4 cups boiling water

Sauté cornmeal in oil or roast in dry pan. Add salt and boiling water. Cook 30 to 35 minutes or until done.

36. Corn Dumplings

      1 cup corn flour
      1 tsp salt
      Small amount of boiling water to form dough

Mix ingredients and knead to form small round dumplings. Drop dumplings into boiling water and remove when done. Serve with Miso Sauce (204), or any other sauce.

37. Corn Croquettes

      1 cup corn flour
      ½ tsp cinnamon (optional)
      ¼ tsp salt
      Boiling water
      Oil to deep fry or pan fry

Mix dry ingredients and add enough water to make dough. Knead. Form croquettes and deep fry or pan fry in a small amount of oil.

38. Crepes de Mais (Corn Pancakes)

      1 cup cornmeal
      1 tsp oil
      ¼ tsp salt
      ¾ cup water

Sauté the cornmeal well in the oil. Combine with other ingredients to make a thin batter. Fry crepes in an oiled skillet until both sides are crisp.

39. Cream of Corn

      1 cup corn flour
      ¼ tsp salt
      3 cups hot water

Mix corn and salt with hot water. Pour into soup stock or miso soup. Simmer, stirring gently until done.

40. Grain Milk Cereal

      1 cup grain milk powder (kokkoh)
      ½ tsp oil (optional)
      5 cups water
      ¼ tsp salt

Sauté grain milk powder in oil or roast in a dry pan until there is a nut-like fragrance. Cool. Add water gradually to prevent lumping. Add salt. Bring to a boil. Lower flame and simmer until thickened. Cook about 30 to 45 minutes. Serve with sesame salt or soy sauce.

41. Grain Milk Soup

    1 cup grain milk powder (kokkoh)
    ½ tsp oil
    10 cups water
    ½ tsp salt
    Soy sauce

Sauté grain milk powder in oil. Cool. Add water gradually to prevent lumping. Add salt and bring to a boil. Lower flame and simmer until thickened. Stir occasionally. Add soy sauce to taste.
   Variations:
   Serve with any whole grain noodle or macaroni.
   Garnish with chopped scallion.

42. Flakes Cooked as Cereal

    1 cup rice, corn, wheat, rye, oats, or mixed flakes
    ½ tsp oil
    ¼ tsp salt
    3 cups boiling water

Sauté flakes in oil. Add salt and boiling water. Cook 30 minutes.

43. Baked Rice Flakes

    3 cups rice flakes
    ½ tsp oil
    4 cups boiling water
    ¾ tsp salt

Sauté flakes in oil. Add boiling water, salt and bring to a boil. Put into an oiled casserole and bake 30 minutes at 450 degrees. This dish may be varied by adding leftover cooked rice, cereal, or vegetables. It is delicious served with Scallion Miso (206).

44. Vegetable Soup with Flaked Corn

    1 onion, cut in crescents
    5 cabbage leaves, cut in 1-inch squares

1 small carrot, cut diagonally
2 tsp sesame oil
5 cups boiling water
2 cups flaked corn
1 tsp salt
1 tsp soy sauce
2 tsp sesame butter

Sauté vegetables in 1 teaspoon oil, add boiling water, and cook for 25 minutes. While this is cooking, sauté the flaked corn in 1 teaspoon oil until transparent. Add salt to soup, then flaked corn and cook until thickened. Add soy sauce and sesame butter; cook 5 minutes. Serves 7.

45. Corn Pudding

2 cups flaked corn
1 tsp oil
1½ to 2 cups boiling water
½ tsp salt
1 egg
1 Tbsp sesame butter

Sauté flaked corn in oil until transparent, stirring constantly. Add boiling water and salt and continue stirring until thickened. Simmer, covered, for 20 minutes. Beat the egg and add to the corn mixture, stirring vigorously. Add sesame butter and cook 5 minutes longer. Put in a mold that has been rinsed in cold water. Serve cool. Pour Sesame Soy Sauce (222 A) over pudding.

46. Flakes Loaf

3 cups mixed flakes (rice, corn, wheat, rye, oats)
3 tsp oil
3 cups water
1 or 2 onions, chopped
½ leek, chopped
2 Tbsp parsley, chopped
1 clove garlic, minced
¾ tsp salt

Sauté flakes in 1 teaspoon oil, add warm water and cook. Sauté onions, leek, parsley and garlic in 2 teaspoons oil and mix with flakes. Spoon into an oiled casserole and pat the top with water. Bake 50 to 60 minutes in a 400-degree oven.

Sauce for Loaf
1 tsp oil
½ cup soy sauce
½ cup water
1 Tbsp kuzu

Heat oil and add soy sauce. Bring to a boil. Add water and boil several minutes. Dissolve kuzu in small amount of cold water. Add to sauce and cook until thick, stirring constantly.

47. Rice Flakes and Fruit

1 cup rice flakes
1 tsp oil
3 cups water
¼ tsp salt
Any fruit in season

Sauté the flakes in oil. Add water and salt. Cook 15 minutes. Add 1 cup of fruit and cook 10 minutes. Place in a casserole or individual custard dishes. Chill and serve.

Noodles

48. Buckwheat Noodles in Soup

> 1 package buckwheat noodles (soba)
> 2 quarts water
> 3 cups cold water

Bring 2 quarts of water to a boil. Add the buckwheat noodles, and when the water boils again, add 1 cup of cold water. Do this three times and then remove the noodles from the stove, cover and let sit for 5 minutes. Drain, rinse with cold water and reserve. To reheat when needed, pour boiling water over the noodles, drain and arrange in bowls.

> **Soup Stock**
> 1 bunch scallions, minced
> 1 tsp oil
> 3 cups water
> 3-inch piece of kombu
> 5 Tbsp soy sauce

Sauté the scallions in oil. Add 3 cups water and kombu. Bring to a boil. Cover and simmer about 15 minutes. Remove kombu and add soy sauce. Bring to a boil, remove from heat. Serve over noodles in bowls.

Variation: Use any soup stock desired, such as recipes 119, 120, and 121.

49. Soba with Tempura

Prepare Buckwheat Noodles in Soup (48) and arrange shrimp or vegetable tempura on top of the noodles. Sprinkle with chopped raw scallions and Toasted Nori (113).

50. Buckwheat Noodles with Fried Bean Curds

> 1 package buckwheat noodles, cooked
> 2 cups Kombu Stock (118 A)
> 2 fried bean curds in ¼-inch slices
> 2 Tbsp soy sauce
> ¼ tsp salt
> 2 scallions in 1-inch pieces

Bring soup stock to a boil, add bean curds, cover and boil 5 minutes. Add soy sauce, salt, and scallions. Bring to a boil and serve immediately with hot buckwheat noodles. Serves 2 or 3.

51. Buckwheat Noodles Gratin

> 12 oz. buckwheat noodles, cooked
> 2 Tbsp oil
> 2 onions, sliced lengthwise in crescents
> 1 small cauliflower, divided into flowerets
> 6 cups water
> 1 tsp salt
> 1 heaping Tbsp shaved bonita (optional)
> 2 Tbsp soy sauce
> 1½ heaping Tbsp kuzu

Heat oil. Sauté onions, then cauliflower in oil; add water. Bring to a boil and lower heat. Cover and cook for 25 minutes. Add salt and bonita. Cook for 10 minutes. Add soy sauce to taste, keeping in mind that the noodles absorb the flavor. Dissolve the kuzu in 5 tablespoons water and add to the vegetables. Cook until thickened. Place cooked noodles in a covered casserole and pour vegetable mixture over them. Bake 30 minutes in a 350-degree oven.

52. Buckwheat Noodles with Béchamel Sauce

> 1 lb buckwheat noodles, cooked
> 2 tsp oil
> 1 carrot, sliced diagonally
> 2 onions, sliced in thin crescents
> ½ small cauliflower, divided into flowerets
> 1 tsp salt

Sauté carrots, onions, and cauliflower in oil. Prepare the béchamel sauce. Mix with the vegetables and add salt. Place cooked noodles in a covered casserole and pour the vegetable mixture over them. Bake 30 to 40 minutes in a 250-degree oven.

Béchamel Sauce
3 Tbsp whole wheat flour
3 Tbsp oil
2½ cups water
Soy sauce and salt to taste

Add flour to hot oil and sauté stirring constantly until lightly browned. Cool, add water, and cook until thick. Season.

53. Sauces for Udon
Udon may be cooked as described in Buckwheat Noodles (48).

A. Clam Sauce
1 clove garlic, crushed
1 Tbsp oil
½ bunch parsley, minced
1 can chopped clams (fresh, if available)
½ tsp salt
Soy sauce to taste
1 package udon, cooked

Sauté garlic in oil, add parsley and sauté for a few minutes. Add clams and clam liquid. Add salt and cook 10 to 20 minutes. Season with soy sauce. Serve over cooked udon noodles.

B. Scallion Parsley Sauce
1 bunch scallions, chopped
½ bunch parsley, chopped
2 tsp oil
½ tsp salt
Soy sauce to taste
1 package udon, cooked

Sauté scallions and parsley in oil, add a little water, and cook until done. Add salt and soy sauce. Mix in a large pot with noodles and simmer to blend the flavors with the noodles.

C. Onion Parsley Bonita Sauce
>2 large onions, sliced in thin crescents
>2 Tbsp chopped parsley
>1 Tbsp oil
>2 Tbsp shaved bonita
>Water
>1 package udon, cooked

Sauté onions and parsley in oil. Add bonita and a little water and cook until done. Add salt and soy sauce to taste. Mix with noodles and simmer to blend flavor.

D. Mock Meat Sauce
>1½ packages udon, cooked
>2 onions, finely chopped
>1 Tbsp oil
>3 Tbsp miso
>½ cup water
>¼ cup bonita flakes or 1½ Tbsp ground dried fish (optional)

Sauté onions in oil until transparent. Dilute miso in water. Add to onions. Add fish and cook about 20 minutes. Mix sauce and cooked udon thoroughly and cook over low flame for about 10 minutes.

54. Buckwheat Noodles with Miso Sauce
>1 heaping Tbsp miso
>4 Tbsp sesame butter
>1 cup water
>1 tsp grated orange rind (optional)
>1 package buckwheat noodles, cooked

Mix miso, sesame butter, and water. Cook over low heat about 15 minutes, stirring occasionally. Add orange rind. Serve over cooked noodles.
Variation: Serve this sauce with grains or vegetables.

55. Buckwheat Noodles in Kuzu Sauce
Prepare any of the Vegetable Sauces with Kuzu (80). Serve over cooked buckwheat noodles.

56. Fried Buckwheat Noodles with Kuzu Sauce
Cook buckwheat noodles and drain thoroughly. Fry in a small

amount of oil. Serve with any of the Vegetable Sauces with Kuzu (80).

57. Udon, Macaroni, Vermicelli, etc.

Treat in the same manner as any of the buckwheat noodle recipes. (See Topical Index.) Adjust cooking time to type of noodle.

58. Whole Wheat Spaghetti with Vegetable Soup

1 lb whole wheat spaghetti, cooked
2 medium onions, minced
2-inch piece of carrot, chopped
6 cabbage leaves, chopped
2 tsp oil
8 cups water
½ tsp salt
¼ cup soy sauce

Sauté onions, carrots, and cabbage in oil. Add water and bring to a boil. Cover and lower heat. Cook 30 minutes. Add salt and soy sauce. Before serving, add cooked whole wheat spaghetti to soup. Bring to a boil and cook 3 minutes.

59. Udon with Cabbage

1 package udon, cooked
1 medium head cabbage, shredded
2 cloves garlic, crushed
1 Tbsp oil
1 tsp salt

Sauté the garlic and cabbage in oil. Cook over low heat with a cover about 30 minutes or until tender. Stir occasionally. Add salt and cooked udon. Mix thoroughly and cook 10 minutes.

60. Udon with Broccoli

1 package udon, cooked
1 bunch broccoli, chopped
2 cloves garlic, crushed
1 Tbsp oil
1 tsp salt

Boil broccoli till tender and drain. Sauté garlic in oil until brown, add broccoli, cooked udon and salt. Cook about 10 minutes.

61. Udon with Azuki

½ cup azuki beans
1½ cups water
¼ tsp salt
1 bunch scallions, chopped
1 tsp oil
1 tsp salt
2½ tsp soy sauce
1 lb udon noodles, cooked

Put azuki beans and water in a pressure cooker on high heat. Bring to full pressure, lower heat to medium low and cook 45 minutes. Remove from heat and allow pressure to return to normal. Add ¼ teaspoon salt. Sauté scallions in oil, stirring constantly. Add ¼ teaspoon salt and soy sauce. Cook for 5 minutes. Mix all ingredients together. Serve warm in winter. In the summer, put in a square pan and refrigerate. Cut in squares to serve.

Additional Noodle Recipe
210. Udon with Miso Sauce

Vegetables

I. Nitsuke Vegetables: Cut vegetables as shown in Cutting Styles (page 128) and sauté, covered, in a little sesame oil with a pinch of salt. Add a little water to cover the bottom of the pan. Cover and cook over low heat. When the vegetables are cooked, add soy sauce to taste. Using these basic directions, the following vegetable dishes may be prepared.

62. Carrot Sesame Nitsuke

    2 carrots, cut in matchsticks
    1 tsp sesame oil
    1 tsp salt
    1 tsp soy sauce
    1½ tsp roasted sesame seeds

Cook per Direction I, adding sesame seeds after soy sauce. Cook an additional 5 minutes, mixing well.

63. Carrot Walnut Nitsuke

    2 large carrots, cut in matchsticks
    3 Tbsp walnuts, roast in a dry pan and grind
    ½ Tbsp oil
    ½ tsp salt
    ½ cup water
    1 tsp soy sauce

Cook per Direction I, adding walnuts after the soy sauce. Cook an additional 5 minutes, mixing well.

64. Carrot Burdock Kinpira

>   2 burdock roots, cut into matchsticks
>   1 carrot, cut in matchsticks
>   1½ tsp sesame oil
>   ¼ tsp salt
>   1 Tbsp soy sauce

Sauté burdock per Direction I until it changes color slightly. (This takes longer than for most vegetables.) Add carrot, sauté slightly, then add water and salt. Cover and cook over low heat. Add soy sauce to taste.

65. Onion Nitsuke

>   2 large onions, sliced lengthwise in crescents
>   2 tsp oil
>   ½ tsp salt
>   Soy sauce

Cook per Direction I. Season with soy sauce.

66. Carrot Onion Nitsuke

>   Carrots, cut in matchsticks
>   Onions, sliced lengthwise in crescents
>   Oil
>   Salt
>   Soy sauce

Prepare according to Direction I.

67. Onion Cabbage Nitsuke

>   Onion, sliced in crescents
>   Cabbage, cut in strips
>   Oil
>   Salt
>   Soy sauce

Prepare according to Direction I.

68. Endive Nitsuke

>   5 endive, cut in half lengthwise
>   2 tsp oil
>   1 tsp salt
>   Soy sauce

Prepare according to Direction I.

69. String Bean Nitsuke

> String beans
> Oil
> Salt
> Soy sauce

Remove tips and stems and cook whole according to Direction I. Season with soy sauce.

70. Broccoli Nitsuke

> 1 bunch broccoli, chopped in small pieces
> 2 tsp oil
> 1 cup water
> ¼ tsp salt
> Soy sauce

Prepare per Direction I. Season with soy sauce to taste.

> **II. Sautéed Vegetables:** Sauté the vegetables in a little sesame oil, with a pinch of salt, stirring constantly until done. No water is added; the vegetables cook in their own juices. Soy sauce may be added to taste at end of cooking. The following dishes may be sautéed in this manner.

71. Sautéed Watercress

> 1 bunch watercress, finely chopped
> 1 tsp oil
> ¼ tsp salt

Sauté per Direction II until liquid is evaporated. 1 tablespoon sesame butter may be added to enhance the flavor.

72. Sautéed Celery with Scallions

> 1 bunch scallions, chopped
> 2 stalks celery, thinly sliced
> 1 tsp salt
> 1 tsp oil

Sauté per Direction II until liquid is evaporated.

73. Sautéed Swiss Chard

      1 bunch swiss chard, finely chopped
      1 tsp oil
      ¼ tsp salt

Sauté per Direction II. This is also very delicious if mixed with Béchamel Sauce (159 A).

74. Sautéed Carrot

      1 carrot, cut in matchsticks
      1½ tsp oil
      ⅛ tsp salt

Sauté per Direction II.

> **III. Vegetables with Miso:** Sauté vegetables, covered, in a small amount of sesame oil with a pinch of salt. Add a little water if necessary and cook covered over low heat until done. Add diluted miso and simmer a few minutes longer.

75. Scallion Miso

      1 bunch scallions
      2 tsp oil
      1 Tbsp miso, diluted with a little water

Mince scallion roots. Cut the rest in small pieces, separating the green parts and the white parts. Sauté the roots, then the green parts and then the white parts. Stir very gently. Add miso and cook slowly over a low flame for 5 minutes, covered. Mix together and cook without cover for 5 more minutes or until fragrant.

76. Onion Carrot Miso

      1 lb small white boiling onions
      1 carrot, sliced diagonally
      2 Tbsp miso
      ½ tsp salt
      1 Tbsp oil

Mince 3 of the onions. Sauté the minced onions, then the remaining whole onions, then the carrot in oil with salt. Add water to cover and cook until vegetables are done. Add miso and cook 5 more minutes.

77. Onion Miso

    5 onions, cut in thin crescents
    ⅛ tsp salt
    1 Tbsp oil
    3 Tbsp miso

Sauté onions in oil with salt. Add miso and simmer 5 minutes, covered. One teaspoon grated orange rind may be added.

78. Vegetable Miso Stew

    4 small onions, whole
    1 daikon radish, cut in large pieces
    2 carrots, cut in 2-inch pieces
    4 small albi, whole (optional)
    2" x 3" piece of kombu
    ¼ tsp salt
    Miso or soy sauce to taste

Cover vegetables with water, and add salt. Cook as long as you wish. The longer you cook it, the more delicious it is. Scallions may be added near the end of cooking, threaded on bamboo skewers or toothpicks so that they hold together. Add miso or soy sauce to taste. Serves 4.

79. Boiled Pumpkin with Miso

    Cut pumpkin into large pieces. Mince onions and sauté in oil. Add pumpkin and continue to sauté. Add water and a pinch of salt. Boil until tender or pressure cook for 20 minutes. Add miso, diluted with water, to taste, and simmer a few minutes longer.

> **IV. Vegetable Sauces:** Sauté vegetables in sesame oil with salt. Add water and cook, covered, until done. Dissolve kuzu, or arrowroot, in cold water and add to vegetables. Cook until thick, stirring constantly. Add soy sauce to taste.

80. Vegetable Sauces with Kuzu

A. Carrot Cabbage Sauce

    2 small carrots, sliced in thin rounds
    ¼ cabbage, thinly sliced
    2 medium onions, sliced lengthwise in crescents
    2 tsp oil
    ½ tsp salt
    3 cups water
    1 Tbsp kuzu or arrowroot
    3 Tbsp cold water
    2 tsp soy sauce

Sauté vegetables in oil with a pinch of salt. Add 3 cups water and salt and simmer 45 minutes or until tender. Dissolve kuzu in 3 tablespoons cold water and add to vegetables. Cook until thick, stirring constantly. Add soy sauce to taste. Serves 4 or 5.

B. Cauliflower Sauce

    2 onions, sliced lengthwise in crescents
    ¼ Chinese cabbage, shredded
    ½ cauliflower, broken into flowerets
    1 carrot, sliced diagonally
    2 tsp oil
    ½ tsp salt
    3 cups water
    1 Tbsp kuzu or arrowroot
    3 Tbsp cold water
    2 tsp soy sauce

    Cook according to Direction IV.

C. Cucumber Sauce

    2 medium onions, sliced lengthwise in crescents
    3 cucumbers, sliced
    ½ carrot, sliced diagonally
    2 tsp oil
    ½ tsp salt
    3 cups water
    1 Tbsp kuzu or arrowroot
    3 Tbsp cold water
    2 tsp soy sauce

Cook according to Direction IV.

D. Carrot Turnip Sauce

1 lb onions, sliced in thin crescents
½ lb carrots, cut diagonally
½ lb turnips, cut diagonally
1 Tbsp oil
1 tsp salt
8 cups water
6 Tbsp kuzu, dissolved in water
4 Tbsp soy sauce

Cook according to Direction IV. Serves 15.

E. Lotus Carrot Daikon Sauce

Lotus root, cut in rounds
Carrot, cut diagonally
Daikon radish, cut in rounds
Oil
Salt
Water
Kuzu, dissolved in water
Soy sauce

Cook according to Direction IV.

F. Turnip Sauce

Turnips
Oil
Salt
Water
Kuzu, dissolved in water
Soy sauce

Leave turnips whole if small or cut in rounds if large. Cook according to Direction IV.

G. Onion Sauce

Onions, cut in crescents
Oil
Salt
Water
Kuzu, dissolved in water
Soy sauce

Cook according to Direction IV.

V. Vegetables with Soy Sauce and Sesame Butter:
Sauté vegetables in a little sesame oil with a pinch of salt. Add a small amount of water and cook, covered, until done. Add equal parts sesame butter and soy sauce mixed with a little water. Cook until mixture coats vegetables.

---

81. String Beans with Sesame and Soy Sauce

Remove tips from string beans and cook whole as described above.

82. Watercress with Sesame and Soy Sauce

Chop watercress finely and cook as indicated.

83. Tempura

Tempura Batter 1
1 cup whole wheat pastry flour
1¼ cups water
½ tsp salt
1 tsp arrowroot flour

Tempura Batter 2
1 cup whole wheat pastry flour
½ tsp salt
1 to 1¼ cups water
1 tsp sweet rice flour

Tempura Batter 3
½ cup whole wheat flour or whole wheat pastry flour
½ cup unbleached white flour
1 egg, well beaten
½ tsp salt
1 cup water

Tempura Batter 4
½ cup whole wheat flour
½ cup buckwheat, rye, or corn flour
½ tsp salt
1 to 1¼ cups water

Mix selected batter lightly. Lumps don't matter. The vegetables and the batter should be chilled. For best results, mix batter just prior to use.

Vegetables are dipped in batter or mixed with batter and deep fried in vegetable oil or sesame oil. The oil should be 3 inches deep and heated to approximately 350 degrees. When the batter-dipped vegetables are added to the oil, they should fall to the bottom of the pan and almost immediately float to the surface. Cook until yellow on one side, turn, and cook until yellow on the other side. Drain well on paper toweling. Serve hot.

Examples of Vegetable Tempura

Carrots—Cut carrots very thinly. Mix with a sufficient amount of batter and drop by spoonfuls into hot oil.

Onion—Cut onions in half lengthwise and slice thinly, leaving a piece of core at the bottom of each slice to hold the slivers together. They should look like fans. Dip into batter and deep fry.

Carrot Onion—Slice carrots thinly and chop onion. Mix with batter and drop by spoonfuls into hot oil.

Watercress—Leave whole and dip one side only in batter.

Cauliflower—Divide into flowerets and dip into batter.

Burdock Root—Sliver, pre-cook, and mix with slivered carrot. Mix with batter and drop by spoonfuls into hot oil.

Lotus Root—Thinly cut in rounds. Use no batter. Pre-salt and place on paper towel to drain. They are like potato chips.

Celery—Chop and use in combination with any other vegetable. The leaves of celery or carrots may be added to other vegetables for variety and color.

Squash or Pumpkin—Thinly slice in approximately 3-inch strips, ¼-inch thick.

Corn—Scrape kernels off cob. Add chopped onions and mix with batter. Drop by spoonfuls into hot oil.

Other—Many other vegetables and combinations may be used.

84. Squash or Pumpkin

These two vegetables may be used interchangeably in any recipe.

A. Baked Squash

Cut squash in large pieces, sprinkle with salt and bake at 350 degrees until soft. Serve with soy sauce or Miso Sauce (204).

B. Boiled Squash

Cut squash in large pieces. Mince onions and sauté in oil. Add squash and sauté. Add water and salt. Simmer, covered, until tender and add soy sauce to taste.

C. Pressure Cooked Squash

Cut squash in large pieces. Sauté minced onion and then squash in pressure cooker. Add a very small amount of water, only enough so that the bottom will not scorch. Bring to full pressure. Lower the heat and cook for about 20 minutes. Bring pressure down by running cold water over top of pressure cooker. Note: The onions may be omitted although they add to the sweetness of the squash.

Variation: Blend and use as filling in pies and muffins.

85. Stuffed Acorn Squash

> 2 carrots, cut in thin rounds
> 3 large onions, finely chopped
> 1 small cabbage, thinly sliced
> 3 or 4 large acorn squash, halved
> 2 Tbsp oil
> 2 tsp salt
> 5 shrimp, thinly sliced (optional)
> 1 cup unbleached white flour or whole wheat pastry flour
> 1½ cups water or more
> 1 egg, beaten (optional)

Cut squash in half lengthwise and trim the bottom side of each half, if necessary, so it will lie flat. In 1 tablespoon oil, sauté onions, cabbage, carrots, and shrimp, in that order, adding one at a time. Cook for about 10 minutes on a medium flame. Salt to taste. In 1 tablespoon oil, sauté the flour and cool. Add about 1½ cups water and ½ teaspoon salt to the flour mixture. Combine this mixture with the vegetables. Add the egg. Oil the edges of the squash. Fill and bake at 450 degrees for 45 to 50 minutes.

86. Corn

A. Boiled Corn

Boil ears of corn in salted water. Serve with soy sauce.

B. Roasted Corn

Leaving husks on but removing silk, wet corn and wrap in the husks, twisting them to cover corn. Coat corn with soy sauce and roast for a few minutes. Roast young ears of corn over a fire or in the oven.

87. Corn Casserole

> 1 cup corn pulp, grated off cob
> 2 eggs, separated
> ½ to 1 tsp salt
> 1 Tbsp oil
> ½ cup bread crumbs or ¼ cup unbleached white flour
> Parsley

Add well-beaten egg yolks to corn, then oil, salt, and bread crumbs. Fold in stiffly beaten egg whites. Mixture should be just stiff enough to drop from spoon. Put in well-oiled casserole or mold and bake in a 350-degree oven in a pan of hot water about 20 minutes or until puffed. Garnish with parsley.

88. Cauliflower

Place whole cauliflower stem down in boiling salted water. Bring to a boil again, cover and let bottom cook and top steam until done, about 7 minutes. Cool, remove leaves and separate flowerets; cut the stem from the bottom and proceed by pulling each floweret apart, cutting stem when necessary.

Variation: Steam the cauliflower in a steamer until tender and prepare in the same manner.

89. Broccoli

Boil broccoli in salted water until bright green or steam in a steamer. Cut as desired. Béchamel Sauce (159 A) may be poured over broccoli.

90. Lotus Root Balls

> 1½ cups lotus root, grated
> 1 cup minced onion
> ½ tsp salt
> 1½ cups whole wheat flour
> Oil for deep frying

Mix the above ingredients well. Form into little balls and deep fry.

Variation: Use carrots in place of lotus root.

91. Lotus Root Balls Béchamel

Prepare Lotus Root Balls (90). Make Béchamel Sauce (159 C or

D). Pour sauce over the lotus root balls and serve.

92. Creamed Onions

>   12 small onions
>   ½ tsp salt
>   1 tsp bonita flakes (optional)
>   2" x 2" kombu
>   2 cups water
>   Béchamel Sauce (159 B)
>   1 tsp grated orange rind (optional)

Pressure cook onions for 3 minutes with the bonita, kombu, salt, and a little water. Reserve the liquid. Make béchamel sauce, using reserved liquid; add orange rind for flavoring. Pour over the onions. Serves 6.

Variation: Prepare Pastry (254). Roll pastry and place in rectangular baking casserole. Pour the creamed onions into pie crust and bake in a 450-degree oven until crust and top are golden.

93. Stewed Vegetables

>   6 small onions, whole
>   6 small or 3 large carrots, cut in half
>   6 string beans, whole
>   6 large pieces of daikon radish, turnip, or any root
>   vegetable
>   6 cups water
>   4" x 4" piece of kombu
>   3 Tbsp soy sauce
>   Salt to taste

Place all ingredients in a large pot and bring to a boil. On very low flame, simmer several hours. The longer it is cooked the better the taste. Serve one piece of each vegetable to each person.

94. Vegetable Buckwheat Casserole

Sauté onions, carrots, and cauliflower in a little oil. Add a little water and simmer. Add salt to taste. Place in a casserole and pour thin Buckwheat Cream (26) over it. Bake in a 350-degree oven for 30 minutes.

95. Vegetable Buckwheat Noodle Casseroles

A. Buckwheat Noodles with Béchamel Sauce

>   1 lb buckwheat noodles, cooked

2 tsp oil
1 carrot, sliced diagonally
2 onions, thinly sliced
½ small cauliflower, divided into flowerets
1 tsp salt
Béchamel Sauce (159 C)

Sauté onions, carrots, and cauliflower in oil. Combine béchamel sauce with vegetables and add salt. Place cooked noodles in a casserole and pour the vegetable mixture over them. Cover and bake 30 to 40 minutes in a 350-degree oven.

B. Buckwheat Noodles Gratin

12 oz. buckwheat noodles, cooked
2 Tbsp oil
2 onions, sliced in crescents
1 small cauliflower, divided into flowerets
6 cups water
1 tsp salt
2 Tbsp soy sauce
2 Tbsp kuzu

Sauté onions, then cauliflower in oil and add water. Bring to a boil and cook over low heat for 25 minutes. Add salt. Cook for 10 minutes. Add soy sauce to taste. Dissolve kuzu in 5 tablespoons water and add to vegetables. Cook until thickened. Place cooked noodles in a casserole and pour vegetable mixture over them. Cover and bake 30 minutes in a 350-degree oven.

96. Vegetable Pie

1 onion, sliced lengthwise in crescents
1 small carrot, halved lengthwise and sliced
3 cabbage leaves, cut in ½-inch squares
½ turnip, cut in half then thinly sliced
2 tsp oil
12 small shrimp (optional)
2 cups water
½ tsp salt
Pastry (253)
Béchamel Sauce (159 C)

Sauté vegetables in oil, add water and shrimp, and bring to boil. Simmer until tender. Add salt. Line pie plate with pastry and flute the edges.

Place vegetable mixture in pie shell and cover with béchamel sauce. Bake in a 450-degree oven for about 45 minutes or until the crust is done.

97. Onion Pie

> 2 small carrots, thinly cut diagonally
> 4 onions, sliced lengthwise in crescents
> 1 Tbsp sesame oil
> 2 eggs, beaten
> ¼ cup unbleached white flour
> 1 tsp salt
> ½ cup water
> 2 or 3 scallions, sliced
> Pastry (257)
> Sesame seeds

Sauté vegetables in oil on high flame. Add salt and water. Lower heat to medium and cook about 15 minutes stirring occasionally. Cool vegetables and add eggs. Add flour and mix well. Line a square baking dish with pastry and flute edges. Put vegetables in the pie shell. Sprinkle with sesame seeds and bake at 450 degrees for 30 minutes.

98. Nagaimo (Cultivated Jinenjo)

A. Deep Fried Nagaimo
Cube small nagaimo into 1-inch pieces. Sprinkle with salt. Deep fry. Drain. Put in a saucepan, add soy sauce, and cook until all the pieces are coated.

B. Nagaimo Patties
Grate nagaimo. Chop onion or scallion and mix with whole wheat pastry flour. Season with salt and form into patties. Use rather large amount of oil in a frying pan, heat the oil, put in the patties, cover and fry until soft and fluffy.

C. Nagaimo Balls
Prepare nagaimo as in B. Drop by spoonfuls into deep oil and fry.

D. Nagaimo Balls in Béchamel Sauce
Prepare Nagaimo Balls (98 C) and make Béchamel Sauce (159 C). Pour sauce over the nagaimo balls.

E. Raw Grated Nagaimo
Grind 1 cup of grated nagaimo in a suribachi. Add ½ cup of soup

stock, 1 tablespoon sake and soy sauce to taste. Grind well. Place in a small dish. Sprinkle with Toasted Nori (113). Serve with soy sauce.

Variation: Mix grated nagaimo with soup stock or in miso soup. Simmer a few minutes.

99. Dandelion Nitsuke

Wash dandelion leaves well. Cut into small pieces. Sauté in oil with a pinch of salt. Add water if necessary and simmer covered until done. Add soy sauce to taste.

100. Dandelion Root

> 1 cup dandelion roots
> 1 Tbsp sesame oil
> Salt and soy sauce

Wash dandelion roots well, do not peel. Cut into thin round pieces. Sauté in oil and season.

101. Miso Vegetable Relish

> ½ lotus root (¾ cup), very finely chopped
> 1 onion (¾ cup), very finely chopped
> ½ burdock (¼ cup), very finely chopped
> ½ carrot (¼ cup), very finely chopped
> ½ cup water
> ¾ tsp grated ginger (omit for sick people and children)
> ¼ cup sesame oil
> 1½ cups miso mixed with ½ cup water
> 1 Tbsp sesame butter

Sauté burdock in sesame oil for 5 minutes. Add onion and sauté, then lotus root and carrots. Add ½ cup water, bring to a boil and cook 5 minutes. Add ginger. Add miso mixed with water. Bring to a boil, lower flame, and simmer 1½ hours, covered. Add sesame butter and cook uncovered for 10 minutes or until the excess water evaporates. This relish may be stored in the refrigerator for a long period of time. Use a small amount on rice, spaghetti, cereals, etc.

Additional Vegetable Recipes
218. String
219. Dried Daikon
223. Vegetables with Sesame Butter Soy Sauce

Beans and Sea Vegetables

Beans: Beans should be picked over and washed thoroughly. Chickpeas and black beans should be soaked several hours. Cook beans in 2½ to 3 times the amount of water for pressure cooking, 4 times the amount of water for regular cooking. Salt should be added only after cooking; if added in the beginning, the beans do not become tender.

---

102. Azuki Beans, Black Beans, Chickpeas

A. Pressure Cooked Beans
½ cup beans
1¼ cup water
⅛ to ¼ tsp salt
½ to 1½ tsp soy sauce

Place beans and water in pressure cooker. Bring to full pressure and cook 45 minutes. Allow pressure to return to normal. Add salt and soy sauce. Cook slowly until liquid boils off. Adjust seasoning to taste.

B. Boiled Beans
½ cup beans
2 cups water
Kombu
¼ tsp salt
Soy sauce to taste

Bring beans and water to boil with a small piece of kombu and cook over low heat for about 2 hours. Add salt and soy sauce and continue to cook without cover over low heat until liquid boils off.

103. Beans with Onions

> 1 minced onion
> 1 tsp oil
> 2 cups beans
> 5 cups water
> 1 tsp salt

Sauté onion in oil. Pressure cook beans, water, and onions 45 minutes. Allow pressure to return to normal. Add salt and cook uncovered until liquid evaporates. Chickpeas and kidney beans are delicious this way.

Variation: Cook beans by any method. Sauté minced onion in oil until cooked but not browned. Add onion to cooked beans.

104. Rice with Beans

> ¼ cup beans
> ¾ cup water
> 2 cups rice, washed
> 3¼ cups water
> ¾ tsp salt

Cook beans in ¾ cup water in pressure cooker for 20 minutes. Let pressure return to normal. Pour off liquid and reserve. Add rice, 3¼ cups water (this measurement should include the reserved liquid from cooking the beans) and salt. Pressure cook 40 minutes over low heat. Remove from heat and allow pressure to return to normal. Mix before serving.

105. Baked Chickpeas with Béchamel Sauce

> 1 cup chickpeas
> 2 onions, minced
> Béchamel Sauce (159 C)
> ¼ tsp salt

Cook chickpeas and onions by any method, reserving cooking water. Prepare béchamel sauce using cooking water from chickpeas. Pour sauce over chickpeas in a casserole and add salt. Bake in a 350-degree oven for 30 minutes.

106. Buckwheat Azuki Pancakes

> 1 cup buckwheat flour
> 1 to 1½ cups water
> ¼ to ½ tsp salt
> ¼ cup azuki beans, cooked

Mix flour, water, and salt to form a thin batter. Pancakes that are too thick have a raw taste. Add beans and stir well. Spoon batter onto a hot greased frying pan and cook as you would regular pancakes.

107. Udon with Azuki Beans

> 1 lb udon noodles, cooked
> ½ cup azuki beans
> 1½ cups water
> ¼ tsp salt
> 1 bunch scallions, chopped
> 1 tsp oil
> ¼ tsp salt
> 2½ tsp soy sauce

Cook noodles and put aside. Put azuki beans and water in a pressure cooker on high heat. Bring to full pressure, lower heat to medium low, and cook 45 minutes. Remove from heat and allow pressure to return to normal. Add ¼ teaspoon salt. Sauté scallions in oil, stirring constantly. Add ¼ teaspoon salt and soy sauce. Cook for 5 minutes. Mix all ingredients with noodles. Serve warm in winter. In the summer, put in a square pan and refrigerate. Cut in squares to serve.

108. Chestnut Azuki Kanten

> 1 cup azuki beans
> 1 cup dried chestnuts
> 5 cups water
> ¾ tsp salt

Pressure cook azuki beans and chestnuts together in 5 cups water for 45 minutes. Add salt. Mash, leaving small pieces.

> 2 bars kanten, small pieces
> 3 cups water
> ½ tsp salt

Break kanten into small pieces and soak briefly in water until softened. Squeeze out water. Add softened kanten to 3 cups water and ½ teaspoon salt. Bring to boil and cook 20 minutes, uncovered. Add chestnut azuki mixture and cook another 10 minutes without cover, reducing the liquids. Rinse mold or serving dish with cold water. Pour mixture into it. Chill in refrigerator. Cut into serving pieces.

109. Chickpea Party Dip

1 onion, minced
1 tsp oil
1 cup chickpeas, soaked
2½ cups water
½ tsp salt
1 Tbsp soy sauce
1 Tbsp sesame butter

Sauté onions in oil. Pressure cook chickpeas with onions and water for 45 minutes. Add salt, blend in a blender until thick and creamy. Add soy sauce and sesame butter and blend again.

110. Deep Fried Kombu

Clean kombu by wiping it with a damp cloth. Cut with scissors into 1" x 4" pieces and tie each piece into a loose knot. Or, cut into 1½" x 3" pieces, slit the center of each piece and pull one end through the slit. Deep fry in 2 inches of oil.

111. Kombu in Soy Sauce

8 oz. kombu
1 qt. soy sauce

Clean kombu by wiping with a damp cloth; cut into 1/2-inch squares. Soak in bowl overnight with soy sauce to cover. Put kombu and soy sauce into a pot, cover, bring to a boil, lower flame and simmer about 3 hours, stirring occasionally. Remove cover and mix thoroughly. Continue cooking and stirring until soy sauce is absorbed. It is extremely salty and only 2 or 3 pieces should be eaten at any one meal. It can be stored in a covered container for many years.

112. Nori with Soy Sauce

1 package nori
2 cups water
3 Tbsp soy sauce

Break nori into 1-inch squares. Soak in water for 20 minutes. Cook in the same water for 30 minutes in covered saucepan. All the water should be absorbed. Add soy sauce, cover, and simmer 30 minutes longer. Stored in refrigerator this will keep for a week or more.

113. Toasted Nori

Roast nori until crisp on one side only over either gas or electric burner of stove. Crush into small pieces. Use as garnish on rice, vegetables, soup, etc.

114. Hijiki Squares

Stuffing
- ¼ cup hijiki
- 2 Tbsp oil
- 4 carrots, cut in matchsticks
- 3 large onions, sliced in thin crescents
- 4 cabbage leaves, chopped
- 4 flowerets of cauliflower, cut in small pieces (other vegetables such as watercress may be used)
- 1 tsp salt
- 3 Tbsp soy sauce

Soak hijiki for 5 minutes. Drain and reserve water. Wash hijiki until clean. Drain and sauté in oil, add remaining vegetables and sauté. Mix in salt, soy sauce, and soaking water. Cook without lid for about 15 minutes until water is evaporated.

Wrappers
- 1½ cups whole wheat flour
- 1½ cups unbleached white flour
- ½ tsp salt
- 2/3 cup water
- 1 Tbsp oil

Mix flours, salt, and water. Add oil, and mix well. Roll into 20 little balls. Roll out each of these balls into very thin 3-inch squares. Spoon portion of stuffing onto a square and cover with a second square. Seal edges with fork or fingers. If stuffing breaks through, seal with kuzu mixed with very little water. Deep fry the packages in oil.

Sauce
- 2 tsp kuzu, dissolved in 2 Tbsp cold water
- 1½ cups water or stock
- Soy sauce to taste

Add dissolved kuzu to water or stock. Simmer until thick. Season with soy sauce. Pour this sauce over the squares as you serve them.

115. Hijiki with Lotus Root

> 3 oz. hijiki
> 8 oz. lotus root (1½" x 2" piece)
> 1 Tbsp soy sauce
> 2 Tbsp sesame oil

Wash hijiki, cover with water, and soak 5 minutes. Strain water and save. Cut hijiki in ½-inch lengths. Cut lotus root in thin slices. Sauté 10 minutes in oil until sticky. Add hijiki, sauté another 5 to 10 minutes. Add soaking water to cover. Bring to boil, add soy sauce and cook 1 hour, uncovered. *Note:* If fresh lotus root is not available, dried lotus root may be used. Soak before using.

Variation: Use burdock or carrot, slivered, in place of lotus root.

116. Kombu Roll

> 2 pieces of nishime kombu (6" x 3")
> 3 cups water (reserve water from soaking of kombu)
> 1 carrot, quartered lengthwise
> 1 burdock root, quartered lengthwise
> 8 strips kampyo, 6 inches long
> 2 Tbsp soy sauce

Soak the kombu in water until it is pliable and easy to handle. Cut the vegetables. Soak kampyo. Place a piece of kombu on a flat surface and arrange the vegetable strips along the length. Roll tightly and tie in four evenly spaced places with the kampyo strips. Repeat for the other roll. Place the rolls in a pressure cooker and add the soaking water to cover them. Cook under pressure for 30 minutes. After pressure goes down, add soy sauce and simmer for 10 minutes. Or, cook in a saucepan for 1 hour, add soy sauce, and simmer another half hour. Cut each roll in 4 serving pieces.

117. Wakame Salad

> 2 cups wakame
> 1½ cucumbers, sliced very thin
> 1 tsp salt
> 2 oranges

Wash wakame and soak in water for 20 minutes. Cut soft leaves from the stems. Save wakame stems for miso soup. Cut leaves in ½-inch pieces. Mix cucumber with 1 teaspoon salt. Let sit for 20 minutes and mix with wakame. Peel the oranges and separate into sections. Remove the skin from each section. Mix orange pieces with wakame. Serve 1 heaping tablespoon per person. Serves 20.

Soups

118. Kombu Stock

A. Plain Kombu Stock

> 3" x 12" kombu, slashed at 1-inch intervals
> 7 cups cold water

Add cold water to kombu, and bring to a boil over medium flame, remove kombu.

B. Kombu Stock with Dried Fish

> 3" x 12" kombu
> 14 cups cold water
> ¾ cup chuba iriko (dried fish)

Bring kombu to a boil in 7 cups water, covered. Add fish, boil again. Strain and reserve kombu and fish. Add 7 more cups water to kombu and fish; cook 30 minutes, covered. Drain; mix with first stock or use separately. Each has a slightly different taste.

119. Clear Broth

> 1 cup Kombu Stock (118A or B) plus 1 cup water
> ½ tsp salt
> 1½ Tbsp soy sauce

Heat soup stock, add salt and soy sauce. Garnish with chopped scallions and/or Toasted Nori (113).

Variations:

Serve buckwheat noodles in the broth. Garnish with sliced scallions and Toasted Nori (113).

Arrange tempura on top of buckwheat noodles.

120. Clear Broth with Vegetables

2 quarts water
1 large piece of kombu
3 onions, sliced
½ lb string beans, carrots, onions, etc.
2 tsp oil
2 tsp salt
½ Tbsp ground Chuba Iriko (187 C), optional
3 Tbsp soy sauce
Chopped scallions
Toasted Nori (113)

Boil kombu in water for 10 minutes. Remove kombu. Sauté onions and string beans until nearly done. Add vegetables, salt and fish to stock and simmer 30 to 45 minutes. Season with soy sauce and sprinkle with scallions and nori. This broth may be served over buckwheat noodles.

121. Clear Broth with Bonita Flakes

3-inch piece of kombu
6 cups water
1 Tbsp bonita flakes
½ tsp salt
2 Tbsp soy sauce

Bring water and kombu to a boil. Remove kombu and add bonita flakes. Bring to a boil and cook one minute. Remove from the stove and allow bonita flakes to settle. Strain and add salt and soy sauce. Reheat and serve as a clear broth or over buckwheat noodles. If used over noodles, more soy sauce may be needed as the noodles absorb the flavor.

122. Other Broths

A. Soy Sauce Vegetable Broth

1 small onion, sliced in crescents
1-inch piece of carrot, cut in matchsticks
3 cabbage leaves, chopped
1 tsp Ground Chuba Iriko (187 C), optional
1 tsp sesame oil
5 cups water
½ tsp salt

3 Tbsp soy sauce

Sauté the vegetables in oil, adding fish powder last. Add water and salt and simmer until vegetables are done. Add soy sauce. Simmer 10 minutes and serve. Serves 5.

B. Soy Sauce Vegetable Stock

2 onions, chopped
1 carrot, chopped
1 tsp salt
12 cups water
4 to 8 Tbsp soy sauce

Put all ingredients except soy sauce in a pot and boil. Reduce heat and simmer 1 hour. Add soy sauce, cook 10 minutes. Strain and serve.

> **Miso Soups**: Because the base of miso is soybeans, miso soup is high in vegetable protein. This soup can be taken every day at one meal.

123. Miso Soup Variations

A. Onion Carrot Cabbage Miso Soup

1 cup minced onion
2 tsp dried fish powder or fish flakes (optional)
2 cups minced cabbage
⅓ cup minced carrot
2 tsp oil
4 cups water
4 tsp miso

Sauté onions, fish flakes, cabbage, carrot in oil, in that order, adding one at a time. Add 4 cups boiling water. Cook 20 to 30 minutes. Dilute miso in a little water, add and simmer 3 minutes. Serve plain or with Toasted Nori (113). Serves 6.

B. Carrot Cabbage Daikon Miso Soup

2-inch piece of daikon radish, cut in small pieces
2 large cabbage leaves, finely cut
1 small carrot, cut in matchsticks
1 tsp oil
5 cups water
5 tsp miso

Sauté radish, cabbage and carrot in oil, in that order, adding one at a time. Add boiling water and cook 40 minutes. Add diluted miso and simmer 3 minutes. Serve immediately.

124. Creamed Miso Soup

> 6 small whole onions
> 3 carrots, cut in ⅓-inch diagonals
> ½ tsp salt
> ⅓ cup whole wheat pastry flour
> 1 Tbsp oil
> 6 cups water
> 2 tsp bonita flakes (optional)
> 2 Tbsp miso

Cook whole onions and carrots in 2 cups water with ½ teaspoon salt under pressure for 7 minutes, or in a saucepan until done but firm. Reserve and cool liquid. Sauté flour in oil, stirring constantly, until it is slightly darkened in color and has a nut-like fragrance. Cool. Put 4 cups of water in a saucepan and add the fish flakes. Boil 5 minutes. Strain and reserve. Make a paste of the flour and the reserved vegetable liquid. Add the paste to the stock to thicken it. Add the vegetables and cook 5 minutes. Add miso and simmer 3 minutes. Serves 6.

125. Root Vegetable Soup with Miso

> 5 scallions, cut in 1½ inch pieces
> 8 oz. salmon or trout (optional), cut in 1 inch cubes
> 1 medium albi, sliced in rounds
> ½ turnip, cut lengthwise in thin crescents
> ½ small daikon radish, quartered lengthwise, sliced thin
> 1 carrot, quartered lengthwise, sliced thin
> 1 Tbsp oil
> 6 cups boiling water
> ¼ tsp salt
> 2 Tbsp miso

Heat oil in saucepan and quickly sauté scallions, fish, albi, turnip, radish and carrot, in that order, adding one at a time. Add 6 cups boiling water and ¼ teaspoon salt. Bring to a boil, cover, lower flame and cook 20 minutes. Dilute miso in a little water and add. Simmer 3 minutes. Serves 6.

126. Vegetable Soup with Flaked Corn

    1 onion, cut in crescents
    5 cabbage leaves, cut in 1-inch squares
    1 small carrot, cut diagonally
    2 tsp sesame oil
    5 cups boiling water
    2 cups flaked corn
    1 tsp salt
    1 tsp soy sauce
    2 tsp sesame butter

Sauté vegetables in 1 teaspoon oil, add boiling water, and cook for 25 minutes. While this is cooking, sauté the flaked corn in 1 teaspoon oil until transparent. Add salt to soup, then flaked corn and cook until thickened. Add soy sauce and sesame butter; cook 5 minutes. Serves 7.

127. Vegetable Soup with Fish and Flaked Corn

    4 small onions, sliced lengthwise in crescents
    1 large carrot, sliced diagonally
    5 cabbage leaves, cut in 1-inch pieces
    1 cup cauliflower flowerets
    1½ tsp oil
    7 cups boiling water
    1 tsp salt
    1 small piece of sea bass, salmon, red snapper, or cod; cut in bite-sized pieces
    3 cups flaked corn, sautéed in 1 tsp oil
    1 Tbsp sesame butter
    Soy sauce

Sauté vegetables in 1½ teaspoons oil. Add boiling water and salt and cook 20 minutes. Add fish and cook 5 minutes. Add sautéed flaked corn and sesame butter and cook until thickened. Soy sauce may be added to taste.

128. Russian Soup

    2/3 cup rice, washed
    3 onions, quartered
    1 large carrot, sliced diagonally
    3 large cabbage leaves, cut in ½-inch squares
    2 tsp oil
    7 cups water
    ¾ tsp salt

Roast rice in a dry pan until browned. In a pressure cooker, sauté onions, cabbage, and carrots in oil until well browned. Add rice and mix well. Add 6 cups water and salt. Bring to full pressure. Lower flame and cook 45 minutes. Allow pressure to return to normal. Add 1 cup water and simmer, stirring occasionally for ½ hour. Soup is quite thick like a porridge.

    Note: If you wish to cook this soup in a regular saucepan rather than under pressure, add the same amount of water, but stir occasionally and add water if necessary. Cook about 2 hours.

129. Vegetable Soup

    8 medium onions, quartered
    1 small cabbage, cubed
    1 stalk celery, chopped
    ½ lb string beans, French cut
    5 carrots, sliced diagonally
    3 Tbsp oil
    10 to 12 cups water
    1 small cauliflower, in flowerets
    6 Tbsp flour
    2 tsp salt

Sauté onions, cabbage, celery, string beans, and carrots in 1 tablespoon oil. Cover with water and cook until tender. Cook cauliflower separately in a small amount of water, covered, and mix with other vegetables when they are tender. Sauté flour in 2 tablespoons oil until flour changes color slightly. Cool. Add broth from soup to make a paste. Add thickening and salt to soup and stir gently. Cook about 30 minutes. Serves 12.

130. Folk Vegetable Soup

    1 daikon radish, shaved
    2 medium carrots, shaved

2 large or 3 small burdock roots, shaved
3 tsp oil
6 cups water
¾ tsp salt
1 small bunch of scallions, chopped
Soy sauce

Cut the radish, carrot, and burdock in shavings, like sharpening a pencil. Sauté burdock, radish, and carrot in oil, in that order, adding one at a time. Cover vegetables with water and cook 1 hour. When half done add salt. When almost done, add scallions and soy sauce to taste.

131. Soybean Soup

9 cups water
3 Tbsp chirimen iriko (optional)
2 medium turnips, cut in small pieces
3 onions, sliced in crescents
1 carrot, sliced diagonally
1 Tbsp sesame oil
1 tsp salt
3 Tbsp soy sauce
½ cup soybeans, soaked overnight, blended until creamy

Bring water to a boil. Add fish and cook 5 minutes. Strain and reserve liquid. Sauté vegetables in oil. Add liquid from fish and cook 25 minutes. Add salt and soy sauce. Bring to a boil and add soybeans and cook 30 minutes without a cover. Serves 15.

132. Egg Drop Soup

1 onion, chopped
1 Tbsp oil
9 cups water
3 Tbsp chirimen iriko (optional)
1 tsp salt
3 Tbsp soy sauce
1 egg, beaten
½ bunch raw scallions, chopped

Sauté onion in oil. Add water and fish. Cook for 20 minutes. Add salt and soy sauce. Bring to a boil and add the egg, stirring until it is cooked. Serve with chopped raw scallions. Serves 15.

133. Whole Wheat Noodle Soup

> 1 lb whole wheat noodles, with boiling water to cover
> 2 onions, chopped
> 2-inch pieces of carrot, cut in matchsticks
> 4 cabbage leaves, chopped
> 1 Tbsp sesame oil
> 8 cups water
> ¾ tsp salt
> ⅓ cup soy sauce

Pressure cook noodles in boiling water to cover for 7 minutes. Let stand 5 minutes, drain and reserve. Sauté vegetables, add 8 cups water and cook for 30 minutes. Add salt and soy sauce. Simmer a few minutes longer. Pour soup over noodles and serve. Serves 7.

134. Sea Vegetable Soups

A. Wakame Miso Soup

> 1 handful of wakame
> 5 cups water
> ⅓ cup bonita flakes (optional)
> 1 Tbsp miso

Soak wakame 10 to 15 minutes in cold water. Reserve water. Remove leaves from the hard stems. Chop stems. Cut the leaves in ½-inch pieces. Add stems to water and simmer 30 minutes. Add leaves and bonita flakes. Cook 5 minutes. Add miso diluted in a little water and simmer 3 minutes. Serves 7.

B. Wakame Onion Miso Soup

> 1 handful of wakame
> 5 cups water
> 1 medium onion, chopped
> 1 tsp oil
> 1 tsp dried fish powder (optional)
> 1 Tbsp miso

Soak wakame 10 to 15 minutes in cold water. Reserve water. Remove leaves from the hard stems. Chop stems. Cut the leaves in ½-inch pieces. Sauté onions and wakame stems in oil. Add water from the soaking and cook 30 minutes after water comes to a boil. Add wakame leaves, fish powder and boil again. Add miso diluted in a little water. Simmer 3 minutes. Serves 7.

135. Vegetable Soup au Polenta

    2 white turnips, cut in large pieces
    2 onions, quartered
    1 carrot, cut diagonally
    1 tsp sesame oil
    6 cups water
    3 heaping Tbsp polenta (coarse cornmeal)
    3 tsp sesame oil
    1 cup water
    1 tsp salt

Sauté vegetables in 1 teaspoon oil. Add 6 cups water. Simmer 30 minutes or until tender. Sauté polenta in 3 teaspoons oil and add 1 cup water. Add to soup and boil slowly over low heat. Season with salt. Add soy sauce to taste and simmer a few minutes longer.

Variation: Use coarse ground millet, millet flour, or corn flour for thickening.

136. Squash Potage

    1 medium squash (acorn, butternut, or banana), cut in
      squares
    4 large onions, quartered
    2 tsp oil
    ¾ tsp salt
    6 cups water, total
    3 Tbsp whole wheat pastry flour
    1 Tbsp oil
    Soy sauce to taste

Sauté onions and squash in 2 teaspoons oil. Add 2 cups water and salt and pressure cook for 20 minutes. Place ingredients in a blender or a food mill and make a purée. To 8 cups of purée, add 3 cups water. Roast the flour in 1 tablespoon oil. Cool. Make a paste with 1 cup water and add this gradually to the squash purée, stirring constantly to prevent lumping. Add soy sauce to taste. Simmer 5 minutes or until thickened.

137. Jinenjo Soup

    Grate jinenjo. Mix with soup stock or miso soup. Simmer a few minutes.

138. Oatmeal Potage

Prepare Rolled Oats (32) and thin as desired with water. Sprinkle with minced parsley or watercress.

Variation: Use wheat flour, grain milk, or buckwheat flour as a base for this potage.

139. Bouillon

½ onion, chopped
1 tsp oil
2 cups water
Soy sauce to taste

Sauté the onion in oil and add water. Simmer until tender and season with soy sauce.

140. French Onion Soup

3 onions, thinly sliced in crescents
1 tsp oil
4 cups Kombu Stock (118) or Clear Broth (119)
Soy sauce to taste
Salt to taste
Croutons or dried bread

Sauté onions in oil. Add soup stock and cook until done. Season with soy sauce and salt and simmer 5 minutes longer. Serve over dried bread or with croutons.

141. Fresh Corn Soup

3 ears of corn, kernels only
1½ onions, chopped
1 tsp oil
4 cups boiling water
½ tsp salt
1 Tbsp kuzu dissolved in 3 Tbsp water

Slice kernels from the cobs, then scrape the cobs with the back of the knife. Sauté onions in oil. Add boiling water and corn. Cook 20 minutes or until tender. Add salt and simmer for 5 more minutes. Add kuzu stirring constantly until thick. If soy sauce is desired for flavoring, use half the quantity of salt and add soy sauce to taste. Serves 5.

Sauces

142. Vegetable Curry Sauce

 2 onions, thinly sliced in crescents
 3 Tbsp oil
 1 carrot, slivered
 1½ tsp curry powder
 1 cup whole wheat pastry flour
 ⅓ lb string beans, cut in 1-inch pieces
 11 cups Kombu Stock (118 A) or water
 1½ tsp salt

Sauté onions in oil until browned. Add carrot, curry powder, and flour. Sauté 10 to 15 minutes, stirring occasionally. In another pan boil string beans. Add string beans to other vegetables. Add stock or water and simmer for 30 minutes. Add salt and simmer a few minutes longer. Serves 10.

143. Vegetable Curry with Fish

 1 large onion, quartered
 2-inch piece of carrot, cut diagonally
 6 string beans, French cut
 Sesame oil
 6 cups water, total
 1 tsp salt
 1 tsp curry powder
 3 heaping Tbsp whole wheat pastry flour
 6 pieces fish, cut in 2-inch squares
 ½ tsp salt

Sauté vegetables in 1 teaspoon oil. Add 5 cups water and simmer 30 minutes. Add 1 teaspoon salt. Separately, sauté curry powder and flour in 2 teaspoons oil. Cool and add 1 cup water. Simmer until thickened. Reserve curry sauce. Salt fish with ½ teaspoon salt and let stand 10 minutes. Dip fish in whole wheat flour and fry in 1 inch of oil. Add fish to vegetables. Before serving, add curry sauce and simmer 5 minutes. Serves 6.

144. Vegetable Stew

Stock
    Leftover chicken or fish bones, organic chicken only
    7 cups water
    ½ tsp salt
    ¼ tsp pepper

    2 small onions, quartered
    Winter squash (twice the amount of onions), cut in 1-inch
        squares
    1 Tbsp sesame oil
    3 heaping Tbsp whole wheat pastry or unbleached white
        flour
    1 cup water

Boil stock ingredients over a low flame 1½ to 2 hours. Reduce to 5 cups, strain. Sauté onions and squash in oil. Add stock and cook until tender. Roast flour in a dry pan, cool, and add water. Simmer 15 minutes and add to vegetables. Bring to a boil and simmer 5 minutes longer.

145. Shrimp Cauliflower Sauce

    8 prawns
    ½ tsp salt
    2 Tbsp oil
    1 medium onion, chopped
    1 cup cauliflower, flowerets
    ½ tsp salt
    4 tsp soy sauce
    4 cups water
    1 Tbsp kuzu dissolved in 3 Tbsp water

Remove shells and veins from prawns. Salt with ½ teaspoon salt and let stand for 10 minutes. Sauté prawns until pink in 2 tablespoons oil. Remove. Sauté onions and cauliflower. Add ¼ teaspoon salt and 2 teaspoons soy sauce. Cover and cook 5 minutes. Add water. Boil 15 minutes. Add ¼ teaspoon salt and 2 teaspoons soy sauce. Add prawns and bring to a boil. Add kuzu and bring to a boil, stirring constantly. Serves 4.

146. Shrimp Curry Sauce

    24 shrimp
    ½ tsp curry powder
    2 Tbsp oil
    ½ tsp salt
    2 cups Kombu Stock (118) or water
    1 Tbsp kuzu dissolved in 3 Tbsp water
    3 scallions, chopped

Remove shells and veins from shrimp. Heat curry powder in oil. Add salt. Stir until smooth. Add shrimp and cook until they turn color. Add stock gradually. Dissolve kuzu and add, stirring constantly until thickened. Cover. Bring to a boil and cook 5 minutes. Add chopped scallions. Serves 6.

147. Scallop Cucumber Sauce

    1½ cucumber, thinly sliced in rounds
    1 Tbsp oil
    20 scallops (1 lb)
    4 cups water and scallop liquid
    ½ tsp salt
    4 tsp soy sauce
    2 heaping Tbsp kuzu dissolved in 6 Tbsp water

Sauté cucumber in oil. Boil scallops in enough water to cover about 3 minutes. Drain, reserving liquid. Add water and scallop liquid to cucumbers and simmer about 15 minutes. Add salt and soy sauce. Simmer 5 minutes. Add kuzu and simmer a few minutes longer adding scallops last. If cooked too long, scallops become tough. Serves 6.

148. Onion Béchamel Sauce

    1 medium onion, thinly sliced in crescents
    2 Tbsp oil
    2 Tbsp whole wheat pastry flour
    1 cup water
    ¼ tsp salt
    2 tsp soy sauce

Heat oil and sauté onions until golden. Blend in flour and brown slightly. Gradually add cold water, stirring constantly. Lower flame and simmer 10 minutes. Add salt and cook 5 minutes. Add soy sauce and simmer a few minutes longer. Delicious served with buckwheat groats or noodles.

149. Sesame Sauce

Roast ¼ cup sesame seeds. Crush until they become oily. A suribachi gives the best results or a blender may be used. Add 2 to 3 tablespoons soy sauce.

150. Miso Sauce

> 1 heaping Tbsp miso
> 3 Tbsp sesame butter
> 1 cup water
> 1 tsp grated orange rind

Mix miso and sesame butter. Add water and cook until creamy. Add orange rind. Serve with rice, macaroni, or vegetables.

151. Miso Salad Dressing

Mix equal amounts of miso and lemon or lime juice and serve over lettuce. It is delicious with boiled lettuce too.

152. Thick Soy Sauce

> 1 tsp oil
> ¼ cup soy sauce
> ¼ cup water
> ½ Tbsp arrowroot starch or kuzu

Warm the oil in a saucepan, add soy sauce, and bring to a boil. Add water and continue to boil several minutes. Dissolve arrowroot in small amount of cold water, add to the sauce, and cook until thick, stirring constantly. Serve with grains or vegetables.

Variation: Add 1 tablespoon ginger juice and serve over fish.

153. Sesame Soy Sauce

> 2 Tbsp sesame butter
> 2 Tbsp soy sauce
> 2 Tbsp water

Mix all ingredients together in a pan and cook, stirring constantly until creamy. Serve over grains or vegetables.

154. Sesame Onion Sauce

> 1 minced onion
> 1 tsp oil
> 1 cup water
> 1 Tbsp sesame butter
> 3 Tbsp soy sauce

Sauté onion in oil until transparent. Add water. Cover and cook about 20 minutes on low heat. Add sesame butter and soy sauce, cover and cook 5 minutes.

155. Mayonnaise Sauce

> 1 egg yolk
> 1 tsp salt
> ⅛ tsp pepper
> 1 tsp lemon juice
> ¾ cup safflower oil

Beat yolk, salt, and pepper. Add a few drops of lemon juice and literally one drop of oil. Mix; then add a little more lemon juice and one more drop of oil, and mix. Add remaining lemon juice and continue adding oil drop by drop gradually increasing the amount until the full ¾ cup of oil is mixed thoroughly into the sauce. Adding oil drop by drop prevents separation.

156. Lyonnaise Sauce

> 1 small onion, minced
> ¼ tsp oil
> 1 Tbsp white wine
> 3 Tbsp Béchamel Sauce (159 A)

Sauté minced onion in ¼ teaspoon oil. Add wine and mix with béchamel sauce. This is delicious served with grilled fish.

157. French Sauce

> 2 Tbsp sesame and safflower oil, mixed
> ½ tsp salt
> ½ tsp lemon, grapefruit, or tangerine juice

Mix ingredients very well until they blend together. The sauce will become a darker color.

158. Salad Dressing

    4 Tbsp safflower or olive oil
    ½ tsp salt
    1 egg yolk
    1 Tbsp tangerine or orange juice or 1 tsp lemon juice

Heat oil. Then cool. Add salt. Beat egg yolk separately and add to oil. Beat all together. When creamy, add citrus juice and mix again.

159. Béchamel Sauce

A. White Sauce

    Unbleached white flour
    Oil
    Water or stock
    Salt

Béchamel sauces are prepared with either 2 parts flour to 1 part oil or 3 parts flour to 1 part oil. The sauce is more delicious prepared in the 2:l proportion, but one may not wish to use that much oil if, for example, a dish such as tempura is served at the same meal. The water or stock quantity used determines the thickness of the sauce (½ cup flour with 3 cups stock makes 1½ cups thick sauce).

    Heat the oil and roast the flour gently, stirring constantly. For white sauce, roast only until the lumps disappear; the color should remain unchanged and the flour powdery. Allow the flour to cool or set the pan of flour in cool water in the sink. Add water or stock to the flour gradually, mixing rapidly. A wire whisk will give good results. Simmer sauce for 20 minutes, stirring often. Add salt to taste and simmer a few minutes longer. Keep the sauce warm over very low heat or in a double boiler until serving time to keep sauce from becoming hard. Note: if sauce is lumpy, smooth it in a blender.

B. Light Sauce

    Whole wheat pastry flour
    Oil
    Water or stock
    Salt

Prepare as White Sauce. Allow the flour to turn color slightly as you roast.

C. Brown Sauce
  Whole wheat flour
  Oil
  Water or stock
  Salt

Roast flour until brown but not burned, about 15 to 20 minutes. It will have a nut-like fragrance. Continue as for White Sauce.

D. Gravy
After cooking fish or sautéing any vegetable, remove the fish or vegetable and add flour to the pan in the proportion of 3 parts flour to 1 part oil or drippings left in the pan. Roast the flour and continue as for White Sauce.

Salads and Pickles

160. Pressed Salad

    2 heads Romaine lettuce
    1 carrot, cut very thinly
    ½ bunch red radishes, cut in thin rounds
    2 tsp salt

Cut lettuce in quarters, open and cut in 1-inch pieces. Mix all ingredients thoroughly with the salt. Place in a Japanese salad press or in a bowl with a plate pressing the salad and a heavy object, such as a rock, on top of the plate. When liquid comes to the top, pour it off. The salad may be eaten immediately, but it is more delicious after 2 or 3 days.

    Variations:
    Cabbage and cucumber
    Cabbage and carrot
    Turnip and carrot
    Cabbage
    Daikon radish and tops
    Onion or scallions, Romaine lettuce and red radish

161. Pickles

A. Daikon Pickles

    1 daikon radish
    1 cabbage
    1 grated orange rind
    2 Tbsp salt

Cut daikon in half and hang outside to dry for 4 days. Slice daikon and cut cabbage in ½-inch squares. Mix daikon, cabbage and orange rind with salt. Press in a salad press and eat after one week.

B. Russian Pickles

    10 small pickling cucumbers, whole

1 green bell pepper, cut in quarters
1 onion, minced
2 cups water
4 to 5 tsp salt

Boil salt and water until salt is dissolved. Cool. Pack vegetables in a glass jar. Add sufficient salted water to cover vegetables. Cover jar and leave at room temperature 5 or 6 days. Refrigerate.

C. Dill Pickles
50 pickling cucumbers
3 stalks dill
2 onions, quartered
12 bay leaves
1 clove garlic
½ cup salt
12 cups water

Place cucumbers in layers in a large jar: 2 rows of cucumbers, dill blossoms, then onions, adding garlic and bay leaf at the top. Repeat until full. Boil the salt and water until salt is dissolved. Cool. Pour over the pickles. Let them stand in a warm room for a few days skimming the top of them when the ferment rises. Place under refrigeration after a few days.

162. Daikon Cucumber Salad
Daikon radish, thinly sliced
Cucumber, thinly sliced
French Sauce (157)
Salt

Place daikon in a strainer and add salt. Mix with the hands. Pour boiling water over this and squeeze out the water. Add salt to the cucumbers and let stand for about 5 minutes until the cucumber becomes soft and the liquid begins to come out. Squeeze the water out of the cucumbers. Mix the two vegetables and add French Sauce. Serve 1½ tablespoons per person. Good with fish.

163. Corn and Cucumber Salad
Halve cucumber lengthwise. Cut cucumber as if you were slicing it thinly, but cut only to within ¼ inch of the cutting board. On each seventh cut, slice completely through the cucumber. Add salt. When the cucumber softens (about 5 minutes), bend it gently. It will look something

like a fan. Boil corn in salt water. Slice kernels from cobs and scrape cobs with back of knife. Sprinkle the corn kernels over the cucumber and add Mayonnaise Sauce (155) or French Sauce (157).

164. Watercress, Onion, and Orange Salad

Arrange watercress attractively on a platter. Sprinkle minced onion over the watercress. Remove the skin from the orange, including the thin white inside skin. Cover onion with orange pieces. Pour a mixture of salad oil and salt on top.

165. Fruit Salad

> Cabbage, chopped
> Salt
> Carrot, thinly sliced
> Apple, chopped
> Tangerine or orange pieces
> Water
>
> French Sauce (157)

Put cabbage in a strainer and sprinkle with salt. Pour boiling water over it. Drain and mix with the remaining ingredients. Add French Sauce (157).

166. Watermelon Salad

> 1 egg, hard boiled
> 1 carrot, thinly sliced
> Water
> 2 Tbsp oil
> ¾ tsp salt
> 1 tsp grapefruit juice
> 1 onion, minced
> 2 cups watermelon, cut in ½-inch squares

Separate egg white from egg yolk. Place egg white in a strainer and press it through. Repeat with egg yolk. Place thinly sliced carrot in a strainer and pour boiling water over it. Mix oil, salt and grapefruit juice. Add minced onion and mix. Add carrot and watermelon, mixing each gently. Place in serving dish decorating the top with egg.

167. Apple Onion Cucumber Salad

> Cucumber, thinly sliced

Salt
Apple, chopped
Onion, minced
French Sauce (157)

Sprinkle cucumber slices with salt and allow to soften 5 minutes. Mix with apple and onion and add French Sauce.

168. Vegetable Fruit Salad

1 small cabbage, shredded
1 large carrot, shredded
1 cauliflower, small flowerets
2 apples, cored and chopped into ¼-inch pieces
1 tsp salt
Salad Dressing (158)

Prepare salad dressing using lemon juice. Pour boiling water over cabbage and carrot. Boil cauliflower. Soak apples in salted water. Mix drained vegetables with salt and dressing and mound attractively on a large platter lined with lettuce.

169. Vegetable Salad

Cut cabbage, onion, cucumber, and carrot as desired. Add salt and vegetable oil.

170. Cabbage Salad

Shred cabbage; add salt and vegetable oil.

171. Cooked Salads

A. Cauliflower Carrot Salad

1 cauliflower
2 tsp salt
3 carrots, cut in rounds
½ cup parsley, chopped
Mayonnaise Sauce (155)

Boil whole cauliflower in salted water; cool and separate into flowerets. Boil carrot for 20 minutes. Mix cauliflower, carrot, parsley and add Mayonnaise Sauce.

B. Spinach Carrot Salad

1 bunch spinach

2 carrots
Sesame Onion Sauce (154/222 B)

Clean spinach and place in boiling salted water, stems down, with no cover. When water comes to a boil again, turn the spinach over in the pot. Boil 5 minutes without a cover. Cool quickly in a strainer letting each spinach strip hang separately over edge of strainer. Cut in 1-inch pieces. Boil carrots separately for 20 minutes. Cut in 1-inch pieces. Prepare sauce and mix with vegetables.

C. Spinach Salad

Prepare spinach as in part B. Add Mayonnaise Sauce (155) with soy sauce.

D. Watercress Sesame Salad

2 bunches watercress
½ cup unhulled sesame seeds
2 tsp soy sauce
2 tsp bonita flakes (optional)

Drop watercress into a large pot of boiling salted water, and boil 5 minutes or until cooked. Squeeze out water and cut into ½-inch lengths. Roast sesame seeds and grind well in suribachi into a paste. Add soy sauce and bonita flakes. Thoroughly mix with watercress.

E. String Bean Sesame Salad

2 cups string beans, sliced
½ cup unhulled sesame seeds
2 tsp soy sauce

Cook string beans in boiling, salted water. Remove and cool. Prepare sesame seeds as in part D, add soy sauce, and mix with string beans.

172. Wakame Salad

2 cups wakame
1½ cucumbers, sliced very thin
1 tsp salt
2 oranges

Wash wakame and soak in water for 20 minutes. Cut soft leaves from the stems. Save wakame stems for miso soup. Cut leaves in ½-inch pieces. Mix cucumber with 1 teaspoon salt. Let sit for 20 minutes and mix with wakame. Peel the oranges and separate into sections. Remove the skin from each section. Mix orange pieces with wakame. Serve 1 heaping tablespoon per person. Serves 20.

Special Dishes

173. Chou Farci

> 1 cup buckwheat groats
> 2 cups water
> ½ tsp salt
> 2 eggs, beaten
> 8 cabbage leaves, whole

This is a country dish of the French buckwheat producing region. Mix buckwheat with water and salt. Beat the eggs. Oil a heavy iron casserole. Place a leaf of cabbage on the bottom, pour a layer of buckwheat mixture over this, and then a layer of egg, and top it off with another cabbage leaf. Alternate in this manner making sure to have a cabbage leaf on top. Cover and bake in a moderate oven for 1½ hours. Remove from casserole by inverting over a platter and cut at the table while hot. Or, serve directly from the casserole. Serve with soy sauce.

174. Piroshki

> Carrots, slivered
> Onions, cut in thin crescents
> Watercress, chopped
> Other vegetables, as desired
> Oil
> Cooked rice
> Pastry (253)

This is an adaptation of a Polish recipe. Sauté vegetables in a little oil. Add cooked rice and salt and sauté. Form small balls of this mixture with your hands, dipping them first in cold, salted water. Roll out pastry and cut into rounds 3 or 4 inches in diameter. Place one rice and vegetable ball on each round of pastry. Fold over and press edges together with a fork. They should look like half moons. Pan fry in a little oil or deep fry.
Variations:

Brush tops of piroshki with beaten egg and bake.
Make small individual pies with these ingredients.

175. Gyoza

> 2 cups whole wheat pastry flour
> 1 cup whole wheat flour
> ½ tsp salt
> 1 cup boiling water
> 1 tsp oil

Mix flours, salt, and boiling water. Knead and add oil. Knead until smooth and shiny. Cover with damp towel while preparing filling.

> **Filling**
> Onion, minced
> Scallions, minced
> Chinese cabbage, minced
> Cabbage, minced
> Oil
> Salt
> Flour or bread crumbs

Sauté vegetables lightly in oil and season with salt. Add a small amount of flour or bread crumbs to absorb liquid.

Roll out dough thinly and cut into rounds 2 or 3 inches in diameter. Holding a round in your hand, place a spoonful of vegetable filling in center, fold over, and press edges together, forming 3 pleats on the top side. Drop gyoza into boiling water and cook until done. Remove with slotted spoon. Serve with soy sauce, soy sauce with lemon juice, or serve in soup.

Variations:
Fill gyoza with vegetables and shrimp, fish, or fowl.
For sick people, make the dough from buckwheat flour.

A. Fried Gyoza
Fry boiled gyoza in a little oil until crisp.

B. Deep Fried Gyoza
Fry boiled gyoza in deep oil until crisp.

C. Baked Gyoza in Sauce
Place fried gyoza in a baking dish. Prepare rice cream, millet cream, or béchamel sauce rather thin. Pour over the gyoza and bake.

176. Gnocchi

This is a version of an Italian pasta dish. Into a quart of boiling salted water, gradually add ¼ pound of fine whole wheat pastry flour, stirring constantly. Cover and turn off the heat. Allow this to swell for about 10 minutes. Pour hot mixture into one or more platters which have been rinsed in cold water. Cool completely. Dough should be ½-inch thick. Cut into squares and brown in a heavy frying pan. Serve with fish sauce or vegetable sauce.

177. Paella

> 2 cups rice
> 5 shrimp, cleaned and de-veined
> 5 scallops
> 1 medium onion, minced
> 1 small carrot, thinly sliced
> ½ tsp salt
> 1 tsp soy sauce
> 1½ tsp oil
> 4 cups boiling water
> ¼ cup fresh peas (optional)

This is a version of a Spanish rice and fish dish. Wash rice and drain. In a heavy skillet, roast the rice in ½ teaspoon oil until golden brown. In another skillet, sauté shrimp and scallops in 1 teaspoon oil and remove from the pan. Sauté onions and carrots in the same pan until lightly browned. Remove vegetables and add water and bring to a boil. Place all ingredients in a casserole, mix and cover. Bake in a 350-degree oven for 1 hour. If desired, 5 minutes before the end of cooking, sprinkle ¼ cup of fresh peas over the top for decoration.

178. Chawan Mushi

> 2-inch piece of kombu
> 2 cups water
> ½ tsp salt
> 1 Tbsp soy sauce
> 1 tsp bonita flakes (optional)
> 2 eggs, beaten
> 1 onion, cut in thin crescents
> 1 small carrot, cut in matchsticks
> Oil

This is a Japanese egg custard served as a soup course. Prepare soup stock by soaking kombu in water for 4 hours. Cook with salt and soy sauce 10 minutes. Add bonita flakes and boil 1 minute. Strain and cool. Add beaten eggs to stock when cool. Sauté vegetables in oil until tender. Put vegetables in the bottom of custard cups (covered ones if possible) and pour the stock mixture over them until ¾ filled. Cover the cups and set them on a rack in a pressure cooker with 1 inch water. Cook 5 minutes under pressure. Or, cook 15 to 20 minutes in a steamer or in the oven in a pan filled with a little water.

Variation: Lotus Root Balls (90), pieces of white meat chicken, or pieces of fish (red snapper, sea bass. etc.) may be added to the vegetables.

179. Rolled Omelette

    2 eggs, beaten
    ⅛ tsp salt
    1 Tbsp Kombu Stock (118)
    1 tsp soy sauce
    2 Tbsp chopped celery leaves or
    2 Tbsp chopped onion and carrot, sautéed
    Oil

This is a Japanese version of the omelette. Mix all ingredients. Heat a little oil in a medium frying pan. Pour mixture into pan and cover. Cook until the bottom is done and the top is set. Gently slip the omelette onto a plate and turn it into the pan again to cook the other side until done. Gently remove it to a plate and allow it to cool slightly. Place the omelette on a bamboo mat or a towel and roll, pressing slightly to help maintain the roll shape. Slice diagonally and serve 2 slices per person along with rice and vegetables.

180. Uosuki

    4-inch square of kombu
    7 cups water
    ½ tsp salt
    ⅓ cup soy sauce
    12 Chinese cabbage leaves, boiled in salted water until
        tender
    1 bunch watercress, dipped in boiling water for 2 minutes
    1 lb fresh fish (red snapper, sea bass, etc.)
    ½ lb scallops or shrimp
    1 bunch scallions cut in ½-inch lengths

1 large turnip cut in half and then in ¼-inch slices
1 package whole wheat noodles, cooked and drained

Uo means "fish" in Japanese. This is like a sukiyaki. Place kombu in water and bring to a boil. Add salt and soy sauce. Strain. Roll watercress in cabbage leaves and cut in 1-inch pieces. Cook small amounts of vegetables, fish, and noodles in broth in a skillet, keeping each separate. Cook about 10 minutes. This dish may be prepared in an electric skillet at the table. In this case, arrange the foods to be cooked attractively on large platters, allowing everyone to cook for oneself. Vary the vegetables and fish as desired.

181. Deep Fried Seafood

A large variety of fish may be used such as: red snapper, bass, salmon, halibut, trout, carp, pompano (cavalla), mackerel, bonita, yellowtail sardines, pike, or grey mullet. Small fish (trout, smelt, fresh water fish, surf-fish, etc.) about 2 to 6 inches long may be used whole, including the head and bones.

A. Coated with Flour

Remove scales and clean fish. Cut fish in pieces or leave whole if small. Sprinkle with salt. Coat with flour and fry slowly in deep oil using medium heat. When crisply done, place fish on platter. Vegetable Sauce (80) or Miso Sauce (204) may be poured over fish.

B. Coated with Flour, Egg, and Bread Crumbs

Clean and scale fish. Cut in pieces if large. Sprinkle with salt. Prepare separate dishes of flour, beaten egg, and bread crumbs. Coat fish first with flour, then egg, then bread crumbs. Fry slowly in deep oil using medium heat. Serve with grated ginger. Good with boiled watercress, cabbage, slivered carrot, etc.

C. Tempura

Tempura Batter 1
1 cup whole wheat pastry flour, sifted, or ¾ cup whole wheat pastry flour and ¼ cup sweet rice flour
1¼ cups cold water
¼ tsp salt
1 heaping tsp arrowroot starch

Tempura Batter 2
1 cup whole wheat pastry flour, sifted
1¼ cups cold water

¼ tsp salt
1 beaten egg (cold)

Blend lightly. Lumps don't matter. Too much mixing causes sticking and bad results. Prepare batter just before you plan to use it; don't let it sit. For fish tempura, use fillets rather than thick large pieces. Cut in 2" x 4" pieces.

Examples of Tempura Preparation

Shrimp—Remove shells from shrimp and sprinkle with salt. Coat with tempura batter. Fry in deep oil until golden on one side, turn over, and fry other side until crisp. Drain fried shrimp in sieve, then on paper toweling. Serve with grated daikon radish and decorate with parsley.

> ### Tempura Sauce
> 2 cups Kombu Stock (118 A)
> 5 Tbsp soy sauce

Mix together and bring to a boil. Serve in individual small bowls. Pieces of tempura are dipped alternately in the sauce and radish and then eaten.

Squid—Remove skin from squid. Score lengthwise and across with knife, cut into 1- or 2-inch pieces. Coat with batter and fry. Serve with Vegetable Tempura (83).

Seafood Vegetable—Use any combination of seafood and vegetables, such as scallops, sliced squid, minced onions, diced carrots, diced abalone, etc. Mix with batter and drop by spoonfuls into deep oil.

D. Other Deep Frying Variations

Fried Trout—Marinate fish for 10 minutes in soy sauce to which grated ginger has been added. Dip in arrowroot powder and deep fry.

Fried Carp—Leave scales on. Sprinkle cleaned fish with salt. Mix arrowroot powder and water. Cut several slits in both sides of fish. Coat fish with arrowroot mixture and deep fry.

Fried Oysters or Clams—Drain and sprinkle with salt. Coat with flour and then with a mixture of beaten egg and bread crumbs. Fry in deep oil. (The egg and bread crumbs are mixed together because of the slippery texture of the oysters or clams.)

Smelt Roll Deep Fry—Prepare smelt by cutting off head. Insert knife into middle of abdomen, open, and take out all intestines. Spread fish out so it looks like a fan and then gently remove bone; leave tail on.

Sprinkle with a little salt, grated lemon rind, and flour. Cut watercress into pieces the width of the smelt and place on fish. Roll fish from head end to tail and put a toothpick through the tail to hold fish together. Roll fish in dry flour and deep-fry. Tail should stick up so fish looks attractive when served.

182. Sashimi

A. Red Snapper
Red Snapper
Daikon radish and carrot, shredded
Horseradish or ginger, grated
Soy sauce

Keep fish chilled until ready to cut. Slice attractively into bite size pieces. Arrange one row on dish, mound shredded radish and carrot beside fish, and place second row of fish on vegetables. Serve with grated horseradish or ginger and soy sauce in small dishes.

B. Tuna
Tuna
Daikon radish and carrot, shredded
Horseradish or ginger, grated
Soy sauce

Buy a long piece of tuna, remove skin and bloody parts. Keep fish chilled until ready to cut. Use only good portion and slice thin. Arrange as in part A.

183. Washed Fish

A. Washed Red Snapper
Red snapper fillets
Salt
Daikon radish and carrot, shredded
Ginger, grated
Soy sauce

Slice fillets thin in large pieces. Sprinkle with salt and place in basket or colander. After 20 minutes, run cold water from faucet over fish slowly. When flesh becomes firm, place on bed of shredded raw radish and carrot. Serve individual portions with soy sauce and grated ginger in small dishes.

B. Washed carp
Prepare as in part A, then dip in ice water until the carp has slightly shrunk.

184. Fish Soups

A. Red Snapper Stew
    2-inch piece of carrot, cut in large pieces
    2 small onions, cut in large pieces
    1 small cabbage, cut in large pieces
    ½ cauliflower
    5 pieces of red snapper, 2 inches square
    2 cups whole wheat pastry flour
    2 tsp salt
    1 Tbsp oil

Sauté vegetables in oil. Add water to cover and simmer. (Because cauliflower breaks up when cooked too long, it can be boiled separately. Add just before the stew is thickened with the flour.) Cut red snapper into bite-sized pieces, fry until crisp in deep oil. Add to vegetables and simmer. Sauté flour and salt with oil until browned; cool and mix with water into a thin paste. Pour this into fish and vegetable mixture and simmer until thickened. Serves 5.

B. Red Snapper Clear Soup
    8 cups Kombu Stock (118)
    Red Snapper
    Scallions
    Croutons or cooked noodles
    Orange rind
    Salt
    Soy sauce

Cut fish into small pieces. Boil quickly and remove. Boil sliced scallions an instant. Strain off liquids from separate boilings and add to stock. Season with salt and soy sauce. Place some of each ingredient into Japanese soup bowls. Add stock. Place a small piece of orange rind into each serving and cover. Clear soups of chicken, duck, shrimp, whitebait, etc., are prepared in the same way.

C. Soup Moule
    Onions
    Oil
    Mussels

White wine
Salt

Dice onions and sauté in oil. Add mussels, which have been thoroughly washed. Add small amount of wine, a little water, and boil over medium heat. When shells open, season with salt.

185. Broiled and Baked Fish

Any fish listed in recipe 181 may be used. Scale fish, except for carp, and clean.

A. Broiled Fish

Use either fillets, steaks, or if the fish is small, use the fish split or whole. Red snapper is very good broiled whole on a skewer. Wrap the fins and tail in wet paper to keep them from burning so the fish will look attractive when served.

B. Baked Fish

Bake whole fish or large pieces. Use one of the following methods:
– Sprinkle with salt and bake.
– Marinate in a mixture of soy sauce and ginger for about 10 minutes, then bake.
– Bake fish until half done. Dip in a mixture of equal parts soy sauce and water and bake until done. The marinade may be thickened with kuzu and served as a sauce with the fish.

186. Boiled Fish

A. Boiled Carp

Carp
Water
Soy sauce

Clean carp but do not remove scales. Mix enough water and soy sauce in the proportion of 5 parts water to 1 part soy sauce, to half cover the fish. Bring liquid to boil and then add fish. Simmer without lid very slowly for 20 minutes. Turn fish and simmer 20 minutes more. Eat fish only, not bones.

B. Boiled Smelt

Smelt
Salt
Soy sauce
Ginger, minced

Clean smelt. Sprinkle with salt. Leave 20 minutes. Rinse with water. Mix 5 parts water to 1 part soy sauce, and add a little minced ginger. Cook fish in this mixture 1½ hours.

C. Small Red Snapper
Clean and slice fish, cut into chunks, including head. Boil in mixture of half soy sauce and half water. If a small piece of fish such as a fillet is used, boil for only a short time. The proportion of soy sauce to water may be reduced.

187. Small Dried Fish
Three of the many kinds of tiny packaged fish are chuba iriko, tazukuri, and chirimen iriko. Chirimen iriko are the smallest of the three. The fish are an excellent source of calcium and may be eaten as an accompaniment to rice or used for soup stock.

A. Deep Fried Small Dried Fish
Good as accompaniment for rice. For children, this preparation is too strong (see part C).

> 8 oz. fish (chuba iriko or tazukuri)
> 6 oz. soy sauce, if you want to keep fish a long time, or 4
>   oz. soy sauce for immediate use
> Oil for deep frying

Deep fry fish to light brown, golden color. Drain. Or, pan fry. Heat soy sauce in pan. Shake fish in the pan until dry. Fish will keep a long time if put in a closed jar.

B. Soup Stocks
Use either chirimen iriko or chuba iriko, as tazukuri are too bitter for soup.

> #### Chirimen Iriko Stock
> 1 onion
> 2/3 cup chirimen iriko
> 7 cups water
> Soy sauce
> Salt

Sauté onion. Add fish and sauté. Add water. Bring to boil. Strain. Add salt and soy sauce to taste.

> #### Chuba Iriko Stock
> 7 cups water
> 3" x 12" kombu seaweed

2/3 cup chuba iriko
Soy sauce
Salt

Boil water and kombu. Add fish. Bring to boil again. Strain and reserve kombu and fish. Add salt and soy sauce to taste.

To make a second stock, add fish and kombu to 7 more cups of cold water. Boil 30 minutes. Strain. Add salt and soy sauce to taste. The first and second stocks mixed together are delicious. Leftover fish may be fed to pets. Kombu may be used in soups or vegetable dishes.

C. Other Uses for Small Dried Fish

Chirimen Iriko—Add to tempura for flavor, or use in nitsuke with cabbage or radish.

Ground Chuba Iriko—Roast in a frying pan and grind into powder for miso soup and other uses.

For Children—Use any of the three kinds of fish. Sauté lightly in a dry frying pan.

— Add to cooked rice. Add a little water and simmer again in covered pot on very low flame for half an hour. Add a small amount of soy sauce. Serve with nitsuke.

— Add to Baked Rice Flakes (43).

188. Abalone Nitsuke

Abalone
Turnips, quartered lengthwise and sliced
Carrots, halved lengthwise and sliced
Oil
Salt
Soy sauce

Remove abalone from shell and slice into small pieces. Sauté abalone with turnips and carrots in oil with a pinch of salt. Season with soy sauce.

Variation: Scallops may be substituted for abalone.

189. Clam Miso

Large clams
Onions, minced
Oil
Miso

Open clam shells and remove clams, or heat clams in a pan of water until shells open and remove clams. Reserve shells and strain clam liquid to remove sand. Sauté minced onion in oil. Thin miso with a little clam liquid and add to onions, making a thick sauce. Spoon half the mixture into half the shells. Place one clam on top of the sauce in each shell and cover with remaining sauce. Broil for a few minutes until lightly browned.

190. Scallop Miso Lemon

> 1 lb scallops
> 4 scallions
> Lemon juice
> Miso

Cut scallops in half or in small pieces. Boil in water to cover for 3 minutes. Reserve liquid. Chop scallions and boil in small amount of water. Place 2 tablespoons miso in suribachi or a bowl. Add juice of a lemon and 2 tablespoons scallop liquid and stir until creamy. Add scallions and scallops. Mix well and serve cold.

191. Carp Soup (Koi-koku)

> 1 whole carp, about 1 lb
> Burdock root, 3 times the volume, after cutting, as carp
> 1 Tbsp sesame oil
> 3 heaping Tbsp miso
> 1 cup used bancha tea twigs and leaves, tied in cotton bag
> Ginger, grated

Clean carp and remove the gallbladder carefully so as not to break it. Do not remove scales. Cut whole fish into half-inch slices. Cut burdock in shavings and sauté in oil. Add carp and cover with water. Put bag of tea in soup and simmer 4 or 5 hours until bones are soft. Remove bag of tea. Thin miso with a little water and add to soup. Simmer one more hour. Serve soup with a pinch of grated ginger on top. Eat everything including the bones. Note: This soup may be pressure cooked for 2 hours or until bones are soft. Allow pressure to return to normal, remove bag of tea, and add miso.

192. Coquilles St. Jacques

> 1 small carrot, finely chopped
> 1 small onion, finely chopped

1 tsp oil
⅛ tsp salt
4 Tbsp water
9 scallops, finely chopped
1 tsp parsley, chopped

Béchamel Sauce
1 Tbsp unbleached white flour
½ cup water
1 Tbsp oil
⅛ tsp salt
1 egg, beaten (optional)

Sauté onion and carrot in oil with salt. Add water and simmer. Add scallops when the vegetables are nearly done. Roast flour lightly in oil. Cool and add water gradually. Simmer 20 minutes. Season with salt and stir in beaten egg. Mix scallops and vegetables with the sauce. Put heaping teaspoons of this mixture in clam shells or in individual ramekins and broil for 3 to 5 minutes. Garnish with parsley. Serves 4.

Variations:
Marinate scallops in 1 teaspoon wine.
Add 1 teaspoon lemon juice to the béchamel sauce.

193. Shrimp Cauliflower Sauce

8 prawns
½ tsp salt
2 Tbsp oil
1 medium onion, chopped
1 cup cauliflower, flowerets
½ tsp salt
4 tsp soy sauce
4 cups water
1 Tbsp kuzu dissolved in 3 Tbsp water

Remove shells and veins from prawns. Salt with ½ teaspoon salt and let stand for 10 minutes. Sauté prawns until pink in 2 tablespoons oil. Remove. Sauté onions and cauliflower. Add ¼ teaspoon salt and 2 teaspoons soy sauce. Cover and cook 5 minutes. Add water. Boil 15 minutes. Add ¼ teaspoon salt and 2 teaspoons soy sauce. Add prawns and bring to a boil. Add kuzu and bring to a boil, stirring constantly. Serves 4.

194. Shrimp with Sesame Seeds

>1 lb raw shrimp, shelled and de-veined
>2 scallions cut into 2-inch lengths
>2 Tbsp oil
>¼ tsp salt
>1 Tbsp soy sauce
>2 tsp roasted sesame seeds

Heat oil, add shrimp, scallions, salt, and soy sauce. Cook, stirring constantly, 7 to 8 minutes or until shrimp are tender. Sprinkle with roasted sesame seeds.

195. Rice Canapes (Sushi)

>Raw tuna
>Eggs
>Clams
>Cooked rice
>Orange juice
>Soy sauce
>Grated ginger

Slice tuna into thin pieces. Beat eggs and make an omelette about ¼-inch thick. Cut into pieces the same size as tuna. Take clams out of shells. Boil in soy sauce for a few minutes. Mix about 1 tablespoon orange juice with each cup of rice. Let rice cool. Place a heaping tablespoon of rice in palm of left hand; with the first two fingers of the right hand, shape rice into cylinder shapes with slightly flattened top surfaces. Place either tuna, egg, or clams on each of the cylinders. Press down with fingers. Arrange attractively on platter. Serve with soy sauce to which a little grated ginger has been added.

196. Sushi Mold

>Raw tuna
>Cooked rice
>Orange juice
>Lotus root, thinly sliced
>Carrots, cut in matchsticks
>Eggs
>Soy Sauce

Slice tuna into thin pieces. Mix about 1 tablespoon orange juice with each cup of rice. Let rice cool. Cook vegetables separately; sauté covered in a small amount of oil with a pinch of salt, add a small amount of water, cover and cook until done. Beat eggs and make an omelette about ¼-inch thick. Cut into pieces the same size as tuna. Wet a rectangular, shallow mold. Arrange fish, fried egg, and vegetables attractively. Cover with about 1 inch of rice. Press down, invert over platter, and unmold. Slice into rectangular pieces. Serve with soy sauce.

Variation: Place prepared rice in individual serving dishes and arrange fish, vegetables, and egg over rice.

197. Seafood Pie

> Pastry (254)
> Béchamel Sauce (159)
> Onions, minced
> Parsley, chopped
> Thyme and garlic, minced (optional)
> Oil
> Mussels, clams, oysters, or other shellfish

Make pie shell and bake until nearly done. Prepare béchamel sauce using juice drained from seafood as part of liquid. Sauté onions and herbs. Add seafood and cook slightly until about half done. This may be a very short time and must be judged carefully. Overcooked seafood becomes dry or tough. Add sauce to sautéed mixture and pour into pie shell. Bake in a 450-degree oven until sauce bubbles and begins to brown.

198. Egg Tempura

Use only fertile eggs from chickens that have been organically fed.

A. Egg Tempura without Batter

Heat deep oil to medium temperature. Break one egg into a small bowl and gently slip egg into the oil. Do not let egg get tough from over-cooking.

B. Egg Tempura with Batter

Prepare Tempura Batter (83-1). Pour a small amount of batter into a small bowl. Break one egg into the batter. Gently scoop batter around the egg and turn the bowl over, letting the egg and batter slip quickly into hot oil. Prepare one egg at a time. The oil should be hot enough to cook the batter, but not to overcook the egg. You may have to try this a few times before it comes out perfectly. It should be something like a poached egg.

199. Sesame Chicken

> 2½ lb frying chicken (organic), cut in pieces
> 2 Tbsp oil
> ¼ cup toasted sesame seeds
> 2 tsp salt
> 1 clove garlic, minced
> 2/3 cup sifted whole wheat flour

Preheat oven to 400 degrees. Oil a shallow baking dish. Brush the chicken pieces with oil. Put sesame seeds, salt, garlic, and flour in a paper bag. Add a few pieces of chicken at a time and shake the bag to coat each piece with the flour mixture. Place chicken in the prepared pan. Bake 50 to 60 minutes or until golden.

200. Fried Chicken

> Chicken (organic), cut in pieces
> ½ cup soy sauce
> ½ cup water
> 1 tsp grated ginger
> Flour
> Salt
> Oil

Marinate chicken pieces in mixture of soy sauce, water, and ginger for one hour. Dust the chicken with a mixture of flour and salt. Brown in skillet in a small amount of oil. Cover and cook over low heat or in a slow oven until tender. For crisp skin, remove cover for the last 10 minutes.

201. Deep Fried Chicken

> Chicken (organic), cut in pieces
> ½ cup soy sauce
> ½ cup water
> 1 tsp grated ginger
> Cracker crumbs
> 1 egg, beaten

Marinate chicken pieces in mixture of soy sauce, water, and ginger for one hour. Dip in cracker crumbs, then in beaten egg, and again in cracker crumbs. Deep fry in hot oil.

Variation: Pan fry until browned. Cover and cook over low heat or in slow oven until tender.

202. Roast Chicken or Turkey

Wash organic chicken or turkey thoroughly and dry with paper towels. Rub inside and outside with salt. Place fowl in a pan and brush soy sauce inside and outside. Allow the fowl to marinate in soy sauce for 2 to 3 hours, turning and brushing occasionally to distribute the soy sauce evenly.

Stuffing
  2 cups rice
  4 cups water
  1 tsp salt
  ⅓ cup onions, chopped
  ⅓ cup celery, chopped
  1 Tbsp oil
  4 cups bread crumbs, toasted
  Ginger, grated
  Almonds, chopped

Roast the rice until golden brown. Add water and salt. Simmer 1 hour. Sauté onions and celery in oil until the onion is transparent but not brown. Combine vegetables and remaining ingredients with the rice. Mix and stuff bird. Truss and bake, breast down, uncovered on a rack in a shallow roasting pan in a 225-degree oven for 10 to 14 hours depending on the size of the bird. Cool slightly before carving.

Miso and Soy Sauce Dishes

> **Miso**: Miso is a paste made with soybeans, salt, and grain, fermented by a special enzyme. Miso is rich in protein because its base is soybeans. It imparts a meatlike flavor. Use only the kind of miso that has been processed without chemicals.

203. Miso Spread

> 1 Tbsp miso
> 3 Tbsp sesame butter

Mix well and use as a spread on bread. Boiling water may be added to make a thinner spreading mixture.
> *Variation:* Add 1 teaspoon grated orange rind.

204. Miso Sauce

> 1 heaping Tbsp miso
> 3 Tbsp sesame butter
> 1 cup water
> 1 tsp grated orange rind

Mix miso and sesame butter, add water, and cook until creamy. Add orange rind. Serve with rice, macaroni, vegetables, etc.

205. Miso Sesame Sauce

> 3 Tbsp sesame seeds
> 2 Tbsp miso

Wash sesame seeds. Roast in a dry pan over medium flame, stirring constantly, until seeds are dry and start popping. Place in a suribachi and grind. Mix thoroughly with miso. Add about 2 tablespoons water or liquid from cooked vegetables.

206. Scallion Miso

 1 bunch scallions, with roots
 1 Tbsp sesame oil
 1 heaping Tbsp miso
 1 Tbsp water

Cut scallions in ⅓-inch pieces, separating green and white parts. Chop roots finely. Sauté roots first, then green parts, then white parts, in oil. Make a paste of miso and water. Add to cooked scallions, being careful not to mash them. Cook over low heat about 5 minutes. Serve on bread or with grains. Delicious with Rice Porridge (14).

207. Miso Salad Dressing

 Mix equal amounts of miso and lemon or lime juice and serve over lettuce. It is delicious with boiled lettuce too.

208. Miso Vegetable Relish

 ½ burdock (¼ cup), very finely chopped
 ¼ cup sesame oil
 1 onion (¾ cup), very finely chopped
 ½ lotus root (¾ cup), very finely chopped
 ½ carrot (¼ cup), very finely chopped
 ½ cup water
 ¾ tsp grated ginger (omit for sick people and children)
 1½ cups miso mixed with ½ cup water
 1 Tbsp sesame butter

Sauté burdock in oil for 5 minutes. Add onion and sauté, then lotus root and carrots. Add ½ cup water, bring to a boil and cook 5 minutes. Add ginger. Add miso mixed with water. Bring to a boil, lower flame, and simmer 1½ hours, covered. Add sesame butter and cook uncovered another 10 minutes or until the excess water evaporates. This relish may be stored in the refrigerator for a long period of time. Use a small amount on rice, spaghetti, cereals, etc.

209. Miso Soup

 2-inch piece of daikon radish, cut in matchsticks
 1 tsp oil
 ¼ head of medium cabbage, shredded
 ½ carrot, cut in matchsticks
 5 cups water
 5 tsp miso mixed with a small amount of water

Sauté radish in oil, add cabbage, and sauté for about 5 minutes. Add carrots, stir quickly, and then add water. Bring to a boil and simmer 30 minutes. Add miso and water and simmer for a few minutes. Serves 7. Note: See recipe 123 for variations of miso soup.

210. Udon with Miso Sauce

 1½ packages udon, cooked
 2 onions, minced
 1 Tbsp oil
 ¼ cup bonita flakes or 1½ Tbsp ground dried fish
 (optional)
 3 Tbsp miso mixed with water to make a thick cream

Sauté onions in oil until golden. Add bonita flakes and cook about 20 minutes. Add miso mixed with water. Add miso sauce to udon in a large pot, mix well, and heat through.

211. Rice Porridge with Miso

 2 cups rice
 12 cups water
 ¼ cup miso

Wash rice. Pressure cook ingredients 45 minutes over low heat or bring to a boil in a heavy pot and simmer 1 hour or longer.

212. Deep Fried Miso Balls

 1 cup whole wheat flour
 ⅛ tsp salt
 1 onion, minced
 1 Tbsp miso
 ½ to ¾ cup water

Mix flour and salt. Add onion and miso to flour. Add water gradually to make a dough. Drop by spoonfuls into hot oil. When golden, remove to a strainer, then place on a platter covered with absorbent paper.

213. Onion Carrot Miso

>3 medium onions, minced
>1 Tbsp oil
>1 carrot, minced
>½ cup water
>¼ tsp salt
>2 Tbsp miso

Sauté onions in oil until golden, add carrots, and sauté briefly. Add ½ cup water and salt and cook about 15 minutes covered. Add miso and continue cooking uncovered over a low flame for another 30 minutes or until much of the liquid has boiled off.

214. Vegetables Miso

>2 onions, cut in 6 crescents
>4 cabbage leaves, sliced
>1 carrot, sliced
>1 Tbsp oil
>1½ cups water
>¼ tsp salt
>1 Tbsp miso

Sauté onions, then cabbage, then carrot. Add 1½ cups water and salt and cook 10 minutes. Add miso and cook another 5 minutes. Sauce may be served with grains or noodles.

215. Tekka

A. Tekka Miso

>5 Tbsp sesame oil
>2/3 cup burdock root, very finely minced
>1 tsp Ground Chuba Iriko (187 C), optional
>¼ cup carrot, very finely minced
>⅓ cup lotus root, very finely minced
>1 tsp grated ginger
>1⅓ cups miso

Sauté in oil in the following order: burdock, fish powder, carrot, lotus root, ginger. Add miso. Cook 2 to 4 hours, stirring frequently until it is as dry as possible. *Note*: Ideally this should be made with hatcho miso.

B. Dandelion Root Tekka
    5 Tbsp oil
    ⅛ cup burdock, very finely minced
    ¼ cup dandelion root, very finely minced
    ⅛ cup carrot, very finely minced
    ⅓ cup lotus root, very finely minced
    ½ cup miso

Sauté in oil in the following order: burdock, dandelion root, carrot, lotus root. Add miso. Cook 2 to 4 hours, stirring frequently, until dry.

> **Soy Sauce**: Soy sauce is a liquid condiment made from fermented soybeans, wheat, and salt. It can be used in all cooking for seasoning; add toward the end of the cooking time for most recipes. Only soy sauce made without chemicals and fermented naturally should be used.

216. Tea with Soy Sauce
Hot bancha tea poured over ½ to 1 teaspoon soy sauce in a cup gives the flavor of bouillon and is a very soothing drink.

217. Soy Sauce Broth
    1 onion, minced
    1 tsp oil
    4 to 6 cups water
    3" x 3" piece of kombu
    10 chuba iriko (optional)
    5 Tbsp soy sauce

Sauté onion in oil. Add water and kombu. Break dried fish into small pieces and add. Bring to a boil and cook 30 minutes. Remove kombu and fish. Add soy sauce. Serve as a broth or over buckwheat noodles with scallions and toasted nori sprinkled on top.

218. String Beans
    1 lb string beans
    1 Tbsp oil
    ⅓ cup water
    ¼ tsp salt
    2 Tbsp soy sauce

Wash the beans, trim, and cut in 3-inch pieces. Sauté in oil, add water, cover, and simmer slowly until nearly done. Add salt and soy sauce. Cook until liquid evaporates.

219. Dried Daikon

> ½ cup dried daikon
> Water to cover
> 2 tsp oil
> ¼ tsp salt
> 2 tsp soy sauce

Cover daikon with water and soak 20 minutes. Squeeze out water, reserving the liquid for later use. Sauté daikon in 2 teaspoons oil over medium heat for 10 minutes. Cover with water from soaking, bring to a boil, lower flame, and cook, covered, about 30 minutes until water is evaporated. Add more water, salt, cover, and cook again until water is almost evaporated. Remove cover, add soy sauce, and stir until it is absorbed.

220. Hijiki Sea Vegetable

> ¼ cup hijiki
> Water to cover
> 2 tsp oil
> 2 tsp soy sauce

Rinse hijiki and cover with water. Soak 10 minutes. Drain and reserve soaking water. Sauté hijiki in oil over medium heat 5 minutes. Cover hijiki with strained soaking water. Cook uncovered. When liquid comes to a boil, add soy sauce, and continue boiling until liquid is absorbed. Serve 1 heaping tablespoon per person.

221. Thick Soy Sauce

> 1 tsp oil
> ¼ cup soy sauce
> ¼ cup water
> ½ Tbsp arrowroot starch or kuzu

Warm the oil in a saucepan, add soy sauce, and bring to a boil. Add water and continue to boil several minutes. Dissolve arrowroot in small amount of cold water, add to the sauce, and cook until thick, stirring constantly. Serve on grains or vegetables.

222. Sesame Butter Soy Sauce

A. Sesame Soy Sauce
   2 Tbsp sesame butter
   2 Tbsp soy sauce
   2 Tbsp water

Mix all ingredients together in a pan and cook, stirring constantly until creamy. Serve over grains or vegetables.

B. Sesame Onion Sauce
   1 onion, minced
   1 tsp oil
   1 cup water
   1 Tbsp sesame butter
   3 Tbsp soy sauce

Sauté onion in oil until transparent. Add water. Cover and cook about 20 minutes on low heat. Add sesame butter and soy sauce, cover, and cook 5 minutes.

223. Vegetables with Sesame Butter Soy Sauce
   Greens, any variety
   Soy sauce
   Sesame butter

Cook any greens by sautéing, steaming, or boiling. Drain. Mix equal parts soy sauce and sesame butter. Mix sauce with greens and cook 5 minutes.

Breads and Snacks

General Instructions

Flour—Many varieties of flour may be used to make bread. It is best to use freshly ground flour for the greatest nutritional value. Any combination of the following flours can be used for variety: buckwheat, whole wheat, rice, oat, millet, cornmeal, rye, and chestnut flour. Whole wheat is used most frequently and makes a delicious loaf of bread when used alone or in combination with other flours. Rye flour is more like wheat than any other flour, except that it fails to hold the leavening agent well and, hence, the the loaf is more dense. Bread made entirely of rye flour is very dark and heavy. Add whole wheat flour to make a lighter loaf that will also rise better. Buckwheat flour is heavier than other flours; therefore, only a small amount is added to bread.

Water—Because flours vary in the amount of moisture they absorb, it is usually impossible to give the exact amount of flour and water required. In general, for all breads sufficient water should be used to make the dough stiff enough to knead. To determine the proper consistency, feel your ear lobe. The dough should feel much the same. When the dough stays together and comes easily away from the side of the bowl, it has been kneaded enough.

Salt—The amount of salt used will depend upon the judgment of the baker. For general use, ¼ teaspoon salt per cup of flour is suggested. However, it is a question of taste, climate, and the variety of flour used. For children, ⅛ teaspoon per cup of flour is recommended.

Oil and Preheating—If oil is desired in the dough itself, it is added to the flour before the water is added. However, it is not necessary to use oil in the bread. Preheat your oven to 350 degrees. Heat the pans for a few minutes, then oil them. Heating the pans will cut down the amount of oil needed.

Shaping—The dough may be free-formed and placed in the oven or it may be pressed into bread pans. Dip your fingers in water and gently smooth out the top of the loaf. With a wet spatula, separate the edge of the dough from the pan. Brush the top with oil for a nice crust.

224. Unyeasted Bread

For health reasons you may prefer to eat unyeasted bread because yeast is sugar based. It is a very easy bread to make. It will not be soft and light because no baking powder or yeast is used. However, it carries the full flavor of the grains and when chewed well is a much sweeter bread than one that uses yeast. It is very delicious when toasted.

> 3 cups flour
> ¾ tsp salt
> 1½ cups water

Mix flour and salt well. Add water gradually, stirring well. Be sure that all the flour has absorbed the water. Place in an oiled bread pan and bake for 1½ hours at 300 to 350 degrees. When baked, remove from the pan immediately and let cool on a rack before slicing. *Note*: Because no two ovens are alike, the heat and time schedule may vary. Experiment. Check the process of baking periodically. You can test whether the bread is done by pressing the outside.

Flour Combinations

1. 2 cups whole wheat flour
   1 cup rice flour

2. 2 cups whole wheat flour
   ¾ cup cracked wheat, soaked for 1 hour
   ¼ cup rice flour

3. 1½ cups whole wheat flour
   1 cup cornmeal or 1 cup cracked wheat, soaked for 1
     hour
   ¾ cup buckwheat flour

4. 1 cup whole wheat flour
   1¼ cup buckwheat flour
   ¾ cup cornmeal

5. 1¼ cup whole wheat flour
   ¾ cup cracked wheat, soaked for 1 hour
   ¾ cup buckwheat flour
   ¼ cup cornmeal

6. 1 cup whole wheat flour
   ¾ cup buckwheat flour
   ½ cup cornmeal
   ¾ cup cooked rice or buckwheat groats (do not add
      additional salt to pre-cooked grains)

7. 2 cups whole wheat flour
   1 cup buckwheat flour
   2 Tbsp raisins

Follow the procedure (224), using the same amounts of salt and water. You can be very creative with these breads and invent other combinations. Sometimes adding cooked nitsuke vegetables to a bread will make an interesting variation.

225. Yeasted Bread

The batter method is the quickest and easiest way to make yeasted bread. The yeast mixture is a batter rather than a dough and requires little kneading or shaping. The yeast batter is quickly mixed and allowed to rise in the mixing bowl.

> Pinch of yeast dissolved in ¼ cup warm water
> 2 cups whole wheat flour
> 1 cup rye, buckwheat, rice, or any other flour
> ¾ tsp salt
> 2 tsp oil
> 1½ cups water

Soften the yeast in warm water and let it stand for 5 minutes. In a large mixing bowl blend the flours, salt, and oil. Add the softened yeast and mix well. Add water gradually, stirring constantly.

Cover the bowl and contents with a warm, damp towel. Let it stand for 24 hours in a warm spot away from drafts. After this 24-hour period, add sufficient flour so that the batter holds together to form a loaf.

Bake in a 350-degree oven for about 1½ hours. Remove from pan immediately. Place loaf on a rack and cool before slicing. Makes 1 large loaf.

226. Onion Rolls

  3 cups onions, sautéed
  4 cups whole wheat flour
  1 cup corn flour
  1 cup buckwheat flour
  2½ cups water
  2 tsp salt
  1 Tbsp oil
  1 egg, beaten
  Sesame seeds

Combine flours, sautéed onions, water, salt, and oil. Knead dough to ear lobe consistency. Roll out dough on a floured board until quite thin and cut into triangles. Shape into crescents by rolling them from the straight end toward the point. Brush the top with beaten egg and sprinkle with sesame seeds. Bake in a 350-degree oven for approximately 30 minutes.

227. Chapati

  1 cup flour (whole wheat or buckwheat, etc.)
  ½ tsp salt
  Water

Blend ingredients together, adding water gradually. Knead the dough until it reaches ear lobe consistency. Roll out dough on a floured board. Cut into squares or circles. Place these on an oiled cookie sheet. Bake in a 350-degree oven until crisp and slightly browned.

228. Puri

  Prepare dough as for Chapati (227). Cut into rounds. Drop into hot oil, one at a time, holding them under the oil until they puff up. Then let them rise to the surface. Turn when one side is golden brown and brown the other side. Remove from oil, drain, and put on paper toweling to absorb excess oil. They can be served as bread with the meal or can be stuffed by poking a hole in one side and filling with cooked vegetables or rice; these are eaten by hand. In India, chapati and puri are eaten every day as staple food.

229. Crackers

Flour (buckwheat, whole wheat, oatmeal, etc.)
⅛ tsp salt per cup of flour
Water

Mix the ingredients and knead to ear lobe consistency. Roll out thin on a floured board. Cut into 2-inch squares and prick with a fork. Bake on oiled cookie sheets in a 350-degree oven until crisp and slightly browned.

230. Cracked Wheat Crackers

½ cup whole wheat flour
½ cup cracked wheat, soaked for 1 hour
1 tsp orange rind
¼ tsp salt
Water

Mix cracked wheat with the flour, orange rind, and salt, adding sufficient water to make a sticky dough. Oil cookie sheet. Take a large handful of the dough and press it onto the sheet about ⅛-inch thick, dipping fingers in cold water occasionally and working the dough to an even thickness all over. Wet a knife and score in squares. Bake in a 450-degree oven until crisp, about 15 minutes. Break apart and serve.

231. Biscuits

2 cups whole wheat flour
1 cup rice flour
¼ cup sesame seeds
1 tsp salt
1¼ cups water

Mix ingredients. Knead well and cut into desired shape. Put a little Miso Spread (203) on the top if desired. Bake on oiled cookie sheets in a 350-degree oven for 45 minutes.

232. Sweet Bread

    4 cups whole wheat flour
    2 cups cornmeal
    2 cups buckwheat flour
    2 cups chestnut flour
    2½ tsp salt
    1 tsp cinnamon
    2 Tbsp oil
    5 cups water
    2 Tbsp raisins

Mix flours, salt, and cinnamon well, add oil and mix again. Add water and raisins and mix until the dough is fairly soft but not sticky. Put dough in an oiled, square baking pan. Brush top with egg yolk if desired. Bake in a 350-degree oven for 45 minutes.

233. Fried Buckwheat Sesame Bread

    ½ cup sesame seeds, lightly roasted
    2 cups buckwheat flour
    ¼ tsp salt
    ½ tsp cinnamon
    2 tsp oil
    ¾ cup water

Combine dry ingredients and add oil. Add sufficient water to make a stiff dough. Knead. Shape into a long roll and cut into thin slices. Deep fry in oil or pan fry with a small amount of oil.

234. Azuki Muffins

    3 cups whole wheat pastry flour
    ½ tsp salt
    2 cups water
    1 cup azuki beans, cooked and mashed

Mix dry ingredients. Add water and mix gently to make a thin batter. Fill a hot oiled muffin tin ⅓ full of batter. Spoon heaping tablespoons of azuki beans onto batter. Add batter to fill the muffin tin. Bake in a 350-degree oven for 45 minutes. Makes 12 muffins.

    Variation: Fill muffins with chopped apple, chestnut purée, squash purée, apple butter, applesauce, nuts, raisins, etc.

235. Corn Muffins

> 2 cups cornmeal
> 2 cups water, boiling
> ½ cup grain milk powder (kokkoh)
> 1 cup flour (whole wheat, buckwheat, millet, etc.)
> ½ tsp salt
> 1 tsp sesame or corn oil

Pour 2 cups boiling water over the cornmeal. Add grain milk powder and 1 cup of flour, salt, and oil. Mix well. Knead thoroughly. Add more water if necessary. Place in oiled muffin tins and bake in a 350-degree oven for 30 minutes. Makes 12 muffins.

236. Rice Muffins

> ½ cup rice, cooked
> 1 small onion and 1 small carrot, chopped
> 1 Tbsp oil
> ½ tsp yeast dissolved in 1 cup lukewarm water
> 2-3 cups whole wheat flour
> ½ tsp salt

Sauté onions and carrots in oil. Purée cooked rice and vegetables in a blender. Dissolve yeast in lukewarm water and add to the mixture. Add flour and salt. Knead until the mixture becomes as soft as your ear lobe. Cover with a damp towel and let stand for 5 to 6 hours. Fill oiled muffin tins and bake in a 350-degree oven for 30 minutes.

237. Buckwheat Muffins

> 3 cups buckwheat flour
> 1 tsp salt
> 1 tsp cinnamon
> 4 cups water
> Sesame seeds

Mix flour, salt, cinnamon; add water, and mix well. Oil a muffin tin and fill with the mixture. Sprinkle with the sesame seeds. Preheat oven to 450 degrees and bake for 30 to 40 minutes.

Sandwich Spreads: Any combination of vegetables may be used as a spread. Add any béchamel sauce to vegetables to make a creamy spread.

---

238. Miso Spread

    1 Tbsp miso
    3 Tbsp sesame butter

Mix well and use as a spread on bread. Boiling water may be added to make a thinner spreading mixture.
    Variation: Add 1 teaspoon grated orange rind.

239. Sesame Butter Soy Sauce Spread

    3 Tbsp sesame butter
    1 Tbsp soy sauce

Mix sesame butter and soy sauce and cook for 5 minutes over medium heat until mixture is creamy.

240. Vegetable Spread

    Carrot, finely chopped
    Onion, finely chopped
    Cabbage, finely chopped
    1 tsp oil
    Salt

Sauté vegetables in oil until very soft. Season with salt and cook a few minutes longer.

241. Vegetable Spread with Shrimp

    Carrot, finely chopped
    Onion, finely chopped
    Cabbage, finely chopped
    Shrimp, cut in small pieces
    Oil
    Salt
    Unbleached white flour
    Water

Sauté vegetables and shrimp in oil. Add salt and flour. Add a little water and mix until blended. Simmer a few minutes.
    Variation: Sauté vegetables and shrimp and add Béchamel Sauce (159 A).

242. Squash or Pumpkin Purée

> 1 butternut squash or 1 lb banana squash
> 4 medium onions, chopped
> Oil
> ½ tsp salt

Slice squash into small pieces. Sauté onions, then squash in oil. Add water to cover and salt. Boil until tender or pressure cook for 20 minutes. Strain through a food mill or blend in a blender.

243. Kidney Bean Spread

Mash or purée cooked kidney beans. Season with salt or soy sauce.

244. Whole Wheat Pancakes

> 1 cup whole wheat flour
> ¼ tsp salt
> ¾ cup water

Mix ingredients well and allow to stand for an hour or more. Make pancakes in any size you desire.

Variation: Fill with nitsuke vegetables, fold over, and serve.

245. Vegetable Pancakes

> 1 cup whole wheat pastry flour
> 2 Tbsp arrowroot starch
> ¼ to ½ tsp salt
> 1 onion, finely chopped
> 1 small carrot, finely chopped
> Water sufficient to mix into a batter

Mix ingredients. Cook pancakes on an oiled griddle. Makes 12 pancakes.

246. Azuki Buckwheat Pancakes

> 1 cup azuki beans, cooked
> 2 cups buckwheat flour
> 2½ cups water
> ¾ tsp salt

Mix ingredients gently. Cook pancakes using an oiled frying pan or griddle.

247. Dessert Crepes

>1 cup whole wheat pastry flour
>¼ to ½ tsp salt
>¼ tsp cinnamon
>1 egg, beaten
>1 cup water

Mix ingredients to make a thin batter. In an oiled, small iron pan, add just enough batter to cover the bottom of the pan. Tip the pan so that the batter runs evenly around the bottom. When the first side is browned and the top is set, turn and brown the other side. Fill with apple butter, or other filling. Makes 8 to 10 crepes.

248. Okonomi Pancakes

>1 cup whole wheat pastry flour
>1 cup water
>¼ tsp salt
>½ cup scallions, finely chopped
>½ cup dried shrimp (optional)
>Sesame seeds

Okonomi means "choice" in Japanese. Mix flour, water, and salt thoroughly. Add scallions and shrimp. Oil skillet lightly and heat. Make pancakes 3 inches in diameter. Sprinkle the top (uncooked side) with sesame seeds. Turn and brush with soy sauce. Serve with sesame seed side up.

>*Variation:* Use any combination of vegetables and dried seafood

249. Crepes de Mais

>1 cup cornmeal
>1 tsp oil
>⅛ tsp salt
>¾ cup water

Sauté the cornmeal well in the oil. Combine with salt and water to make a thin batter. Fry crepes in an oiled skillet until both sides are crisp.

250. Buckwheat Crepes

 1 cup buckwheat flour
 3 cups water
 1 egg (optional)
 ¼ tsp salt

Mix ingredients. Heat and oil a small pan. Pour in a thin layer of the mixture and fry on both sides. Remove from pan and fold in quarters. Mound crepes attractively on a plate.

 Variations:

Before folding, fill crepes with nitsuke vegetables.

Fill crepes with chestnuts, raisins, applesauce, or apple butter and serve as dessert.

251. Waffles

 ½ cup buckwheat flour
 ½ cup water
 1 egg, separated
 2 tsp oil
 ¼ to ½ tsp salt

Mix flour and salt. Add water, oil and beaten egg yolk and mix well. Fold in egg whites, which have been stiffly beaten. Bake in an oiled waffle iron.

Desserts

252. Dessert Pastry

     3 cups whole wheat pastry flour
     3 Tbsp oil (corn, a mixture of corn and sesame, or saf-
        flower)
     ½ tsp salt
     1 tsp cinnamon
     1 tsp grated orange rind
     1 cup cold water to form dough

Mix dry ingredients, then work in oil with fingers. Sprinkle with water, a little at a time, and toss with a fork. Add only enough water to moisten dry ingredients and form dough. Roll out thinly on floured board. Makes two 9-inch pie crusts.

253. Pastry I

     3 cups whole wheat flour
     ½ tsp salt
     3 Tbsp oil
     Cold water to form dough

Proceed as in recipe 252.

254. Pastry II

     1½ cups whole wheat flour
     1½ cups whole wheat pastry flour
     ½ tsp salt
     3 Tbsp oil
     1 cup cold water

Proceed as in recipe 252.

255. Pastry III

> 1½ cups whole wheat pastry flour or whole wheat flour
> 1½ cups unbleached white flour
> ½ tsp salt
> 3 Tbsp oil
> 1 cup cold water

Proceed as in recipe 252.

256. Pastry IV

> 3 cups whole wheat pastry flour
> ½ tsp salt
> 3 Tbsp oil
> 1 cup cold water

Proceed as in recipe 252.

257. Kneaded Pastry

> 4 cups whole wheat pastry flour
> ¾ to 1 tsp salt
> 4 Tbsp oil
> 1⅓ cups boiling water

Mix dry ingredients well. Add oil and mix thoroughly. Add water and knead well. Roll out thinly using unbleached white flour to keep dough from sticking to rolling pin and board. This dough may be used for cookies, karinto, chapati, puri, etc.

258. Squash Pie

> Dessert Pastry (252)
> 4 medium onions, cut in crescents
> 1 large butternut squash or 1 lb banana squash,
>   thinly sliced
> ¾ tsp salt
> Water
> Egg yolk (optional)

Sauté onions first, then squash. Add salt and sufficient water to prevent burning. Simmer until tender or pressure cook for 20 minutes. Strain through a food mill or blend in a blender. Pour into pie crust. Put top crust on pie, flute the edges and slash center for steam to escape. Brush top with beaten egg yolk and bake in a 450-degree oven until lightly browned and crisp, approximately 40 minutes.

Variation: After squash is poured into pie shell, one or two diced apples may be placed on top before adding the top crust.

259. Apple Pie

> Pastry (252, 254, 255, or 256)
> 7 apples, thinly sliced
> 1 tsp cinnamon
> ½ tsp salt

Fit pastry to pie pan. Line with apples and sprinkle with salt and cinnamon. Place top crust on pie, flute edges, and slash center. Bake in a 450-degree oven for 30 to 40 minutes.

260. Squash Chestnut Pie

> Pastry (252, 254, 255, or 256)
> 1 cup dried chestnuts
> Water
> Salt
> 1 large butternut squash or 1 lb banana squash, thinly
>   sliced

Pressure cook chestnuts in 2½ cups water for 45 minutes. Salt to taste and simmer uncovered 10 minutes. Purée in food mill or blender. Sauté squash. Add ½ teaspoon salt and sufficient water to prevent burning. Simmer until tender or pressure cook for 20 minutes. Purée in food mill or blender. Fit pastry to pie pan. Pour in squash purée first, then chestnut purée. Cover with top crust, flute edges, and slash center for steam to escape. Bake in a 450-degree oven for 40 minutes.

261. Chestnut Apple Pie

> Pastry (255)
> 1 cup dried chestnuts; 2½ cups water; salt to taste for
>   chestnut purée (260)
> 3 apples, sliced
> ¼ tsp cinnamon
> ¼ tsp salt

Prepare chestnuts as in recipe 260. Fit pastry to pie pan. Line crust with chestnut purée. Place apples on top and sprinkle with ¼ teaspoon salt and cinnamon. Cover with top crust or lattice work crust. Bake in a 450-degree oven for 30 minutes.

262. Sweet Potato Chestnut Pie

    2 large sweet potatoes, peeled and sliced
    1 cup water
    ¼ tsp salt

Cook sweet potatoes in a covered saucepan with water and salt for 20 minutes. Mash or grind in a food mill. Reserve liquid for crust.

    Pastry (252, 254, 255, or 256), prepared with sweet
        potato water
    ¾ cup dried chestnuts
    ⅛ tsp salt
    1½ cups water

Pressure cook chestnuts with water and salt for 45 minutes. Grind half the amount in a food mill. Combine ground chestnuts, whole chestnuts, and sweet potato mixture. Pour into crust, add top crust, and bake in a 450-degree oven for 40 minutes.

263. Apple Strudel

    Pastry (255) using whole wheat pastry flour, double
        recipe
    7 apples, thinly sliced
    1 tsp cinnamon
    ½ tsp salt
    Egg yolk (optional)

Roll pastry into a large circle. Place apples on the pastry, keeping slices separate. Sprinkle salt and cinnamon over apples. Roll carefully, seal edges and brush with egg yolk. Place in oiled baking pan and bake in a 350-degree oven for 45 minutes.

264. Chestnut Roll

    Pastry (257), double recipe
    1 cup dried chestnuts and 1 cup fresh chestnuts, or 2
        cups dried chestnuts
    5 cups water
    Salt
    2 Tbsp chopped nuts

Pressure cook chestnuts in 5 cups water for 45 minutes. Salt to taste and simmer uncovered 10 minutes. Purée in food mill or blender. Roll pastry into a rectangle. Place chestnut purée on pastry and sprinkle with chopped nuts. Roll up and seal the edges. Oil the rolled dough for crispness and place on an oiled cookie sheet. Bake in a 350-degree oven for 45 minuter.

265. The Twist

Filling
1 cup dried chestnuts
1 cup azuki beans
5 cups water
¾ to 1 tsp salt
4 cups apples, chopped
1 Tbsp yannoh (grain coffee)

Pressure cook azuki beans and chestnuts together in 5 cups water for 45 minutes. Add salt. Boil with cover off to reduce remaining liquid. Mash or blend in blender. Cool and add chopped apples and yannoh.

Pastry
5 cups flour
½ to 1 tsp salt
5 Tbsp oil
2 cups boiling water
Egg (optional)

Mix dry ingredients well, add oil, and mix thoroughly. Add water and knead well. Divide dough into 2 balls. Roll out each ball of dough into a rectangular shape and fill each with azuki chestnut mixture. Roll up and seal the edges. Place the 2 rolls in a V-shape, attach and twist together. Brush with beaten egg or oil. Bake in a 350-degree oven for 45 minutes.

266. Apple Crisp

4 cups sliced apples
1 tsp grated lemon rind
⅓ cup whole wheat pastry flour
1 cup rolled oats, uncooked
½ tsp salt
1 tsp cinnamon
¼ cup oil

Place apples in an oiled, shallow baking dish, sprinkle with lemon rind. Combine dry ingredients. Add oil, mixing until crumbly. Sprinkle crumb mixture over apples. Bake in a 350-degree oven for 30 minutes or until apples are tender.

Variation: Use sliced peaches in place of apples.

267. Baked Apples

Core apples, leaving bottom intact. Fill with any one of the following:

> A pinch of salt
> A mixture of sesame butter and salt
> Raisins and salt
> Coarsely grated orange rind and cinnamon

Bake in a 350-degree oven for 30 to 40 minutes.

Variation: Prepare Pastry (256) and wrap apples in the dough. Decorate tops with pieces of pastry in the shapes of leaves or flowers. Brush with egg yolk and bake in a 350-degree oven for 30 minutes or until done.

268. Apple Sauce

Choose flavorful apples such as Delicious, Golden Delicious, Jonathans, or Winesaps. Wash and quarter the apples. Pressure cook 5 minutes with a little salt and just enough water to keep them from burning. Or if prepared in a saucepan, cook until soft. Strain soft apples through a food mill.

269. Apple Butter

Place apple sauce in a large heavy pot and cook uncovered over low heat for 3 to 4 hours or until dark brown and very thick.

270. Apple Chestnut Sauce

> 1 cup dried chestnuts
> 2½ cups water
> Salt
> 3 cups apples, quartered

Pressure cook chestnuts with 2½ cups water for 45 minutes. Salt to taste. Purée half of cooked chestnuts in blender or food mill. Cook apples until soft with a pinch of salt and just enough water to prevent burning. Purée through a food mill. Mix whole chestnuts, puréed chestnuts, and apples.

271. Halvah

> 1 cup whole wheat pastry flour
> 2 Tbsp raisins
> 2 tsp cinnamon
> 1 apple, chopped
> 2 Tbsp sesame seeds
> 1 Tbsp oil
> ½ tsp salt
> 3½ cups water

Sauté flour in oil in a deep skillet. When flour is slightly browned, put aside to cool. Then add chopped apple, raisins, sesame seeds, water and salt. Cook over low heat for about ½ hour, or until thick. Cover skillet and simmer slowly for ½ hour, mixing occasionally. Add cinnamon. Serve hot or pour mixture into a casserole which has been rinsed in cold water. Refrigerate. Unmold and serve. Serves 6.

272. Azuki Pudding

> ½ cup azuki beans
> 2½ cups water
> ⅓ tsp salt
> 1 heaping tsp kuzu

Pressure cook azuki beans in 2½ cups water for 45 minutes. Add salt to taste. Dissolve kuzu in 3 Tbsp cold water and add to beans. Simmer, stirring constantly until thick. Place in wet pan, let cool and refrigerate.

273. Chestnut Azuki Kanten

> 1 cup azuki beans
> 1 cup dried chestnuts
> 5 cups water
> ¾ tsp salt

Pressure cook azuki beans and chestnuts together in 5 cups water for 45 minutes. Add salt. Mash, leaving small pieces.

> 2 bars kanten, small pieces
> 3 cups water
> ½ tsp salt

Break kanten into small pieces and soak briefly in water until softened. Squeeze out water. Add softened kanten to 3 cups water and ½ teaspoon salt. Bring to boil and cook 20 minutes, uncovered. Add chestnut azuki mixture and cook another 10 minutes without cover, reducing the liquids. Rinse mold or serving dish with cold water. Pour mixture into it. Chill in refrigerator. Cut into serving pieces.

274. Kanten Jello

2 bars of kanten
4 cups water
3 cups fruit, in season
Salt

After washing kanten, break into water, and soak for 20 minutes. Cook 15 minutes. Add fruit and cook about 15 minutes. Salt to taste. Strawberries, cherries, melon, or any fruit in season may be used as well as raisins.

275. Rice Pudding

3 cups cooked rice
1 egg
1 cup thin grain milk or water
½ to 1 tsp salt
1 Tbsp raisins
1 tsp cinnamon
⅛ tsp nutmeg

Beat the egg and mix with rice. Add remaining ingredients, mix and place in a casserole. Sprinkle top with nutmeg. Bake in a 350-degree for 30 minutes.

276. Coffee Pudding

1 cup whole wheat flour
1 tsp oil
3 cups water
¼ tsp salt
2 Tbsp yannoh (grain coffee)
1 tsp cinnamon
3 Tbsp hazel nuts, almonds, or walnuts

Sauté the flour in oil until it is lightly browned and fragrant. Cool. Add water, salt and yannoh. Cook until thickened. Add cinnamon and nuts. Serve hot or pour into a casserole that has been rinsed in cold water and refrigerate. Unmold and serve.

277. Rice Flakes and Fruit

    1 cup rice flakes
    1 tsp oil
    3 cups water
    ¼ tsp salt
    Any fruit in season

Sauté the flakes in oil. Add water and salt. Cook 15 minutes. Add 1 cup of fruit and cook 10 minutes. Place in a casserole or individual custard dishes. Chill and serve.

278. Plain Cookies

    1 cup whole wheat pastry flour
    1 cup rice cream powder, roasted
    2 Tbsp sesame seeds
    ½ tsp salt
    2 Tbsp oil
    Water

Mix dry ingredients, add oil, and mix well. Add small amount of water to make a dough that can easily hold together. Roll 1 teaspoon of dough in the palms of your hands. Place on cookie sheet. Flatten if desired. Bake in a oven for 30 minutes.

279. Oatmeal Cookies

    1 cup whole wheat pastry flour
    ½ cup rolled oats, uncooked
    1 Tbsp sesame seeds
    ½ tsp salt
    1½ Tbsp oil
    Raisins, chopped (optional)
    Nuts, chopped (optional)
    Water

Mix dry ingredients. Add oil, raisins, and nuts. Mix well. Add water to make a dough that may be dropped by a spoon onto an oiled cookie sheet. Bake in a 350-degree oven for 30 minutes.

280. Chausson

Prepare Pastry 253, 254, 255, or 256. Knead, roll out thinly, and cut in rounds or squares. Place raisins, apples, and nuts, or Béchamel Sauce (159 A), raisins, and nuts on one-half of each round or square.

Fold over, pinch to seal, and brush with egg yolk. Bake in a 350-degree oven until golden.

Variation: Pastry may be made using a variety of flours and cut and baked as plain cookies.

281. Sand Cookies

Dough
6 cups whole wheat pastry flour
1 tsp salt
2 tsp cinnamon
6 Tbsp oil
2½ cups water

Filling
1½ cups chestnut flour or 1½ cups mashed chestnuts
½ tsp cinnamon
¾ tsp salt
1½ cups water (omit if using mashed chestnuts)
1 apple, chopped
½ cup walnuts, chopped

To prepare dough, mix dry ingredients, add oil, and blend well. Add water and form dough. Separate into 2 balls. Roll one ball to ⅛-inch thickness. Oil a rectangular baking pan and line it with dough. Mix filling ingredients and pour into lined pan. Roll remaining dough. Cover filling, seal and flute edges. Slash top for steam to escape. Brush with beaten egg if desired, and bake in a 450-degree oven for 30 minutes. Cut into squares.

282. Shells

A. Fried Shells
Make Pastry (252). Wrap a strip of thinly rolled pastry around a tubular metal or ceramic mold or stick. Fry in deep oil, cool, and pull out mold. Fill with apple butter (269), chestnut purée (260), or squash purée (260).

B. Baked Shells
Cut Pastry (252) into strips about 1½ inches wide and 4 inches long. Wrap strip around cone shaped mold. Bake in a 350-degree oven until crisp. Fill with apple butter (269), chestnut purée (260), or squash purée (260).

283. Karinto

>1 cup flour (whole wheat or a combination of ½ whole
>   wheat and ½ any other flour such as buckwheat or
>   corn)
>⅛ to ¼ tsp salt
>1 tsp sesame seeds or ¼ tsp cinnamon
>½ cup water

Mix dry ingredients and add water to make pastry. Mix well. Place on
a floured board and knead for 10 minutes. Roll out very thinly and cut
in 2" x 5" rectangles. Cut a 2-inch slit, lengthwise, in the center of each
rectangle and pull one end completely through the slit. Or, cut in any
design you wish. Deep fry in hot oil.

284. Donuts

>5 cups whole wheat pastry flour
>2 cups chestnut flour
>1 to 1½ tsp salt
>1 tsp cinnamon
>⅛ tsp nutmeg
>¼ cup corn oil
>1 egg, beaten
>2 cups raisin water (boil raisins and drain)
>½ tsp grated lemon rind
>½ tsp yeast softened in ½ cup warm water

Mix dry ingredients and sift. Add oil. Mix egg, raisin water, lemon rind,
and yeast. Combine with flour mixture. Knead well and cover with a
damp cloth. Allow to double in size. Roll to ½-inch thickness and cut in
donut shapes. Cover and allow to rise. Deep fry in oil.

Beverages

285. Roasted Green Tea (Bancha)
Twigs and leaves should be choice 3-year-old growth picked from the lower branches of the bush. Roast a handful of twigs and leaves in an unoiled pan over medium heat until lightly browned, not black. Stir constantly as burning occurs easily. Cool and store in a canister. In about 3 cups of water (24 ounces), boil a generous pinch of tea for 10 minutes. Strain and serve. Often several pots of tea can be made from the same leaves by adding fresh water and boiling again.

286. Mu Tea
Boil 1 Mu Tea bag in 4 cups of water for 10 to 20 minutes. Remove tea bag and reserve as it may be used a second time. Mu Tea contains ginseng and 15 other medicinal plants and is considered to be very Yang.

287. Ohsawa Coffee (Yannoh)
This is a grain coffee. Stir 1 heaping tablespoon into 2 cups of cold water. Bring to a boil, remove from the heat until it settles. Simmer for 10 minutes, strain and serve. A few grains of salt added will enhance the flavor. If a coffee entirely free of grounds is desired, strain through cheesecloth.

288. Dandelion Coffee
Wash and dry dandelion roots. Cut into small pieces. Brown in an unoiled pan over medium heat. Cool. Grind in a coffee grinder or mill. For each serving, boil 1 teaspoon dandelion coffee in 1 cup of water for 10 minutes. Strain and serve.

289. Rice Tea
Wash and dry brown rice. Roast, stirring constantly, in an unoiled

pan over medium heat until a rich golden brown. Cool and store in an airtight container until used. For each serving, boil 1 tablespoon of roasted rice in 2/3 cup of water for 20 minutes. Strain. Season with salt and serve.

Note: the strained rice grains may be used as a cereal by adding water and cooking to desired consistency.

Variation: Mix roasted rice with roasted bancha and make tea by boiling in water.

290. Wheat Tea

Wash and dry ½ to 1 cup whole wheat berries. Roast in a dry pan over medium heat until nicely browned. For each serving, boil 1 heaping tablespoon roasted wheat in 2 cups of water for 20 minutes. Strain, salt to taste, and serve.

Note: Wheat may be used as a cereal by adding water and cooking to desired consistency.

291. Grain Milk (Kokkoh)

This is a finely ground combination of roasted rice, sweet rice, oats, and sesame seeds, often used as a milk substitute. Use 1 heaping tablespoon grain milk to 1½ cups of water. Stir and boil for 10 minutes. Serve hot or cold. It is a delicious snacktime pick-me-up.

292. Mugwort Tea

Pick 1 ounce of mugwort leaves. Wash and boil in 1 cup of water about 10 minutes. Salt to taste. Dried mugwort leaves may also used to make tea.

293. Mint Tea

Prepare as Mugwort Tea (292). A stronger flavor is obtained if leaves are bruised with a spoon while cooking.

294. Tea with Soy Sauce (Sho-ban)

Place 1 tsp soy sauce in tea cup, add 2/3 cup boiling bancha tea, and serve. This tea sometimes is used to relieve fatigue.

295. Buckwheat Tea

Save the cooking water from buckwheat noodles. Add salt and soy sauce to taste.

296. Salted Plum Juice (Umeboshi)

Boil 1 salted plum in 2 cups water, simmering gently for about an hour. Strain and serve. For an excellent summer drink, refrigerate and serve cold. It helps quench thirst.

Seasonings

Sea Salt—Sea salt should be used in all recipes calling for salt because it contains trace minerals. Use sea salt that has not been chemically treated.

Gomashio—Sesame salt used at the table in place of plain salt for seasoning on rice, noodles, etc. It has a nut-like salty flavor.

> ¾ cup unhulled sesame seeds
> 1 Tbsp sea salt

Roast the salt in a dry pan and grind to powder in a suribachi. Wash the sesame seeds well. Roast the seeds over a medium flame, stirring constantly with the right hand and shaking the pan frequently with the left hand, until they are slightly toasted and begin to pop. It is very important to roast them evenly so that they all will grind well. Gently grind the sesame seeds and the salt together until 75% of the sesame seeds are crushed, and the salt is coated with the oil of the seeds. Store in an airtight jar.

> *Note*: For children, use a ratio of 1 cup unhulled sesame seeds to 1 tablespoon sea salt.

Umeboshi—Japanese salted plums used in rice balls and in sauces and beverages. They are very salty, not sweet.

Sesame Butter—Ground, roasted, unhulled sesame seeds used in sauces, spreads, and dressings.

Sesame Seeds—Whole, unhulled sesame seeds are used for flavor or decoration.

Ginger—A widely used flavoring, especially good in fish dishes for balance. It also lessens the fish smell.

Cinnamon—Used as a sweetening and flavoring agent in desserts. It is considered to be a most yang spice.

Grated Orange Rind—Used for flavor in desserts, salad dressings, and spreads.

Sesame Oil—Recommended for general use. Especially good for sick or weak people. A more yang oil.

Safflower Oil—Good for dressings and deep frying. A more yin oil.

Note: Those who desire less oil may reduce or omit it from most of the recipes.

Cutting Styles

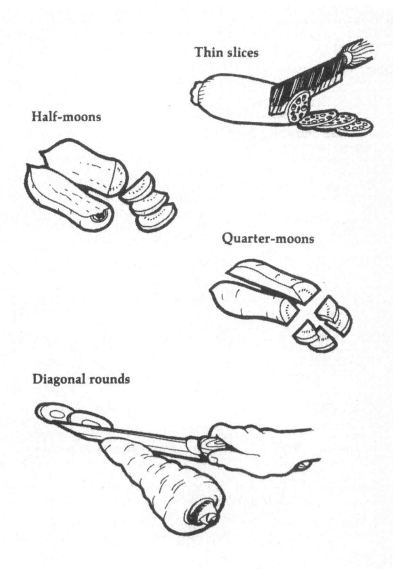

Thin slices

Half-moons

Quarter-moons

Diagonal rounds

Shaved

Matchsticks

Crescents

Minced

Cabbage strips

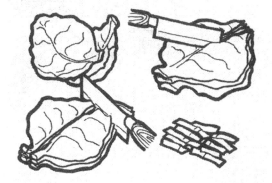

Quartering and slicing

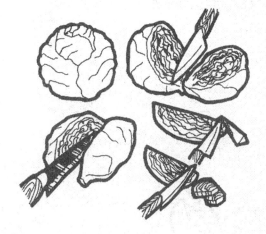

Glossary

Albi (also Satoimo or Taro)—Oriental root vegetable or tuber, similar to a small potato, with a sticky interior.

Azuki—Small, dark red bean.

Bancha—Japanese roasted green tea.

Béchamel—Sauce made by roasting flour in oil and adding liquid. Common in French cooking.

Bonita—Dried and shaved fish used for soup stock or condiment.

Bulghur—Precooked cracked wheat, common in Middle Eastern cookery.

Chapati—Flat wheat bread, a staple of India.

Chawan mushi—Japanese custard made with egg.

Chirimen iriko—Small dried fish used for soup stock, tempura, nitsuke, vegetable pancakes.

Chuba iriko—Small dried silver fish.

Daikon—Long white Japanese radish.

Dashi—Soup stock made with kombu seaweed or kombu and dried fish.

Dashi kombu—Thick kombu used for making dashi, or soup stock.

Gomashio—Common Japanese condiment of sesame seeds and a small amount of sea salt, roasted and ground together.

Gyoza—Pan-fried dumplings stuffed with vegetables.

Hijiki—A dark Japanese sea vegetable of the brown algae family, rich in calcium and iron.

Jinenjo—Wild mountain potato of Japan.

Kampyo—Edible dried gourd strips, often used for tying foods.

Kanten—Seaweed gelatin, also called agar-agar or Ceylon moss.

Kasha—Cooked buckwheat groats, Russian-style.

Kinpira—Sautéed burdock dish, seasoned with soy sauce.

Koi koku—Traditional Japanese stew made with carp and burdock.

Kokkoh—Grain cereal or grain milk made from rice, sweet rice, oats, and sesame seeds.

Kombu—Japanese sea vegetable of the brown algae family, often used for soup stock, nitsuke, and condiments.

Kuzu—High quality starch similar to arrowroot, extracted from the root of a Japanese plant, used medicinally and also in cooking as a thickener.

Miso—Paste made from fermented soybeans, salt, and barley or another grain. Often used as a soup base concentrate.

Mochi—Pounded, steamed sweet rice made into glutinous cakes.

Mugi—Barley.

Nagaimo—Cultivated jinenjo.

Nishime—Cooking style. Vegetables are cut in fairly large pieces, cooked slowly, and seasoned with soy sauce.

Nitsuke—Cooking style. Vegetables are cut fairly small and cooked for a short time.

Nori—Sea vegetable of red algae family, cultivated in Japan and available in thin sheets.

Polenta—Cornmeal.

Puri—Deep-fried puffed dough, often filled with vegetables as a staple sandwich in India.

Sake—Japanese rice wine.

Sashimi—Raw fish.

Sesame Butter—Paste made by grinding roasted unhulled sesame seeds. Good for spreads, sauces, and dressings.

Shiso—Beefsteak leaves.

Shoyu—Soy sauce.

Soba—Traditional Japanese buckwheat noodles.

Sukiyaki—A type of vegetable and noodle dish often cooked at the table.

Suribachi—Ceramic bowl with grooves on the inside used for grinding seeds and other foods.

Suricogi—Wooden pestle for use with suribachi.

Sushi—Cooked rice flavored with citrus juice, umeboshi vinegar, or rice vinegar, often rolled with other ingredients in sheets of nori and served cold.

Tahini—Paste made by grinding hulled sesame seeds. Less nutritious than sesame butter.

Tamari—Liquid obtained in miso making, used in Japan as a thick sauce.

Tazukuri—Small dried blue fish.

Tekka—Condiment made by cooking minced root vegetables with miso until crumbly and dry.

Tempura—Style of cooking batter-dipped foods in deep hot oil.

Tofu—High protein cheese-like cake made from soybeans. Bean curd.

Udon—Large, flat white or whole wheat noodles, often served in soup.

Umeboshi—Japanese plums pickled with salt and beefsteak leaves (shiso), used for seasoning and also medicinally.

Wakame—Kelp-type sea vegetable, native of Japan, often used in miso soup. Leaves are very tender.

Yang—Contractive, having a contractive nature or effect. Opposite of and complementary to yin.

Yannoh—Grain coffee made with roasted and ground rice, wheat berries, chickpeas, azuki beans, and chicory root.

Yin—Expansive, having an expansive nature or effect. Opposite of and complementary to yang.

Recipe Index

Other Books from the
George Ohsawa Macrobiotic Foundation

Acid Alkaline Companion - Carl Ferré; 2009; 121 pp; $15.00

Acid and Alkaline - Herman Aihara; 1986; 121 pp; $9.95

As Easy As 1, 2, 3 - Pamela Henkel and Lee Koch; 1990; 176 pp; $6.95

Basic Macrobiotic Cooking, 20th Anniversary Edition - Julia Ferré; 2007; 275 pp; $17.95

Basic Macrobiotics - Herman Aihara; 1998; 198 pp; $17.95

Book of Judo - George Ohsawa; 1990; 150 pp; $14.95

Calendar Cookbook - Cornellia Aihara; 1979; 160 pp; $24.95

Cancer and the Philosophy of the Far East - George Ohsawa; 1981; 165 pp; $14.95

Cooking with Rachel - Rachel Albert; 1989; 328 pp; $12.95

Essential Ohsawa - George Ohsawa, edited by Carl Ferré; 1994; 238 pp; $12.95

French Meadows Cookbook - Julia Ferré; 2008; 275 pp; $17.00

Macrobiotics: An Invitation to Health and Happiness - George Ohsawa; 1971; 128 pp; $11.95

Naturally Healthy Gourmet - Margaret Lawson with Tom Monte; 1994; 232 pp; $14.95

Philosophy of Oriental Medicine - George Ohsawa; 1991; 153 pp; $14.95

Pocket Guide to Macrobiotics - Carl Ferré; 1997; 128 pp; $6.95

Unique Principle - George Ohsawa.; 1976; 128 pp; $14.95

Zen Macrobiotics, Unabridged Edition - George Ohsawa, edited by Carl Ferré; 1995; 206 pp; $9.95

A complete selection of macrobiotic books is available from the George Ohsawa Macrobiotic Foundation, P.O. Box 3998, Chico, California 95965; 530-566-9765. Order toll free: (800) 232-2372. Or, see *www.ohsawamacrobiotics.com* for all books and PDF downloads of many books.